*The body is your temple.
Keep it pure and clean for the soul to reside in.*

— B.K.S. Iyengar, Yoga Master

Kristy—
Hope you enjoy the book!

Good Luck
& God Bless You!

Scott McGee
May 2003

Or do you not know that your body is the temple of the Holy Spirit who is in you, whom you have from God, and you are not your own? For you were bought at a price; therefore glorify God in your body and in your spirit, which are God's.

— Corinthians 6:19-20

Your Body,
EATING AND EXERCISE FUNDAMENTALS
Your Life™

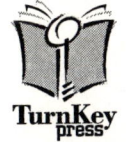

SCOTT McTEER
CSCS, CPT

Your Body, Your Life™

Copyright © 2003 by Scott McTeer.

All rights reserved. No part of this book may be reproduced or transmitted in any form or by any means, electronic or mechanical, including photocopying, recording or by any information storage and retrieval system, without permission in writing by the publisher.

Library of Congress Cataloging-in-Publication Data
McTeer, Scott

ISBN: 0-9740030-6-9

First Edition.

Published in the United States by TurnKey Press

2525 W. Anderson Lane, Suite 540
Austin, Texas 78757
Tel: 512.407.8876
Fax: 512.478.2117
E-mail: info@turnkeypress.com
Web: www.turnkeypress.com

Design by Gestalt Design Studio
Cover Photo Copyrignt © by Paul Traves, F-16 Photography

All Scripture quotations are taken from the
New King James Version of the Holy Bible.

The Your Body, Your Life™ Program is for informational purposes and is not intended to be medical advice. Please consult with your physician before starting any fitness or diet program.

Your Body, Your Life™
EATING & EXERCISE FUNDAMENTALS

by Scott McTeer, CSCS, CPT

Ten Percent of all YBYL™ profits will be donated to church and community organizations.

Possible YBYL™ Program Benefits:

- More muscle tone
- Less body fat
- Optimum body weight and composition
- Less bloating and water retention
- Healthier, younger skin
- Increased metabolism
- Increased utilization of dietary fat
- Improved bone strength
- Increased muscular strength, endurance and flexibility
- Fewer injuries
- Higher quality of life
- More energy
- Better moods
- Less stress, burnout and anxiety
- Greater work performance, productivity and mental acuity
- Greater self-confidence
- Better sleep
- Reduced risk of coronary artery disease and Type 2 diabetes
- Increased good cholesterol and decreased bad cholesterol
- Decreased arterial buildup
- Lower blood pressure
- Lower resting heart rate
- Increased heart volume
- Lower mortality rates
- Decreased incidence of some cancers

Have I not commanded you? Be strong and of good courage; do not be afraid, nor be dismayed, for the Lord your God is with you wherever you go.

— Joshua 1:9

www.ybyl.com

Acknowledgments

First and formost, I thank God for His love and grace.

MY FAMILY
Mom and Dad - Thanks for your love and support. I love you both very much.
Doyal, my brother - You are an inspiration. I love you Susan, Candace and Ryan.

MY BUSINESS PARTNERS & SUPPORTERS
Melanie Meyer, Jo Anne Iaciofano, Katy Powell, Amy Lemen, Chip Conk, C.T., Marion Grant, Sheila Cheng, Ryan Myers and Phenix & Phenix Literary Publicists - Thanks for your guidance, support and knowledge.

MY GREAT COACHES AND MENTORS
Thanks to Coach K for inspiring me to become a great coach.
Thanks to Dr. Gerald Mann at Riverbend Church.
Thanks to Johnny Dawkins and the Duke basketball staff, Quin Snyder and the University of Missouri basketball staff, Dr. Lance Watson, Dr. James Loehr, Dr. Jack Groppel, Pat Etcheberry, Brian Tracy, Jack Shore, Bunner Smith and my dad.
Thanks to Jim Benn for teaching me how to lift weights.

BUSBY'S TOTAL FITNESS (WWW.BUSBYSFITNESS.COM)
Thanks to one of the best gyms in Austin and their "Gym Dogs": Bacchus, Clyde, Roxy, Sam, Matti, Lucy, Maverick, Tasha and the big gym dog, Don.

THE GREAT PERSONAL TRAINERS AT BUSBY'S TOTAL FITNESS
Thanks to: Casey Neuwirth, Keith Busby, James Garland, Terry Tilton, Tom Mixon, Kimberlie Dykeman, Adam Davila, Theo Thurston, Duc Dinh, Connie and Don Busby, John Seay, Michael Schaeffer, Stewart & Sharon Johnson, Todd Essary, Randall Watts, Philip Truong, Resa Chandler, Gianina Garner, Sharon Geller, Binu Sugunan, Craig Johnson, Melissa Benes, Carey Thiel, Shelli Kozenberg, Erica Landon, Jennifer Grosz, Susan Perry, Chase Etcheverry, Chika Christenson, Traci Waters, Christine Tomko, Katrina Waters, and Teresa Pickler.

MY GREAT CLIENTS
You're the reason this book exists: Duke Men's Basketball, University of Missouri Men's Basketball, Lori and Chip Conk, Connie Busby, Greg Crouch, Dawn Stone, Chris Conk, Joellyn Conk and Mike Shannon, Julianne and Matt Lyons, Andrianna and Rob Kelly, Tracy and Bart Sherman, Marion and Dr. Grant, Shelley and Kenny Van Zant, Carol and John Lynch, Karen Spencer, Michael Metteuer, Claudia Mouer, Melissa Muench-Miller, Rob Ellis, Sheila Cheng, Alan Buhler, Jan Daley, Joanne Stewart, Katy Miller, Holly Jacques, Vicki and Mark Collins, Colleen and Kelly Brown, Missy and David Peoples, Janis Tonn, Kristi Tonn, Elizabeth Schmidt, George Farmer, Kristi Mills, Mary Beth Auld, Jennifer Cantu, Suzanne Tieszen, Sandy Lara, Kierra Rycaj, Kristina Mikulencak, Ronnie Ringness, Sherry Smith-Wagner, Brent Wysocki, Nina Bradley, Tom Schoonover, Craig Duke, Curba Lampert, Jane Flynn, Ronnie Ringness, Laurie Frenzel, Peggy Hendricks, Lynn Settles, Kim Waugh, Mary Ellen Brown, Janna Fain, Lisa Becker, Amy Maxson, Amy Brueggeman, Mary Dietz, Beau Leboeuf, Dana Colville, Meetesh Karia, Randy Frazier, Keith Buchanan, Robbie Allen, Raegan Stearns, Sherri and Robert Cooper, Amy Neuenschwander, Jess Christiansen, Michelle Feaver, Lara Mandy, Beverly D, Kirk Rice, Anthony Tatu, Garland Turner, Sara Gates, Nancy Harper and Kazuyoshi Hayashi.

What Scott's Clients Say! YBYL™ Testimonials:

Scott, thanks for being on our team. You've been a big help!
- **MIKE KRZYZEWSKI (COACH K),** DUKE MEN'S HEAD BASKETBALL HEAD COACH

Scott, I've just finished reading your book and think it's fantastic. It's a great motivating, achievement-oriented book that's straightforward and easy to understand and implement. You've done a great job on this ... very well done!
- **JAY BILAS,** ESPN BASKETBALL COMMENTATOR

Scott, I can't tell you how much I appreciate all your support and kindness. You have proven to me that in just one year anything's possible. Your strong words of encouragement and enthusiasm are what keep me motivated. Thank you again for everything you have done to change my life. We make a great team together.
- **ANDRIANNA KELLY,** OWNER, STRAND SALON

Scott's program has had a major positive impact on my health and work. Improving my eating habits and committing to three hours of weekly fitness training is one of the best investments I've made.
- **MATHEW LYONS,** ATTORNEY, ANDREWS & KURTH

Hopefully parents become wiser when they start learning health, fitness and nutrition fundamentals from their children.
- **BOB McTEER,** PRESIDENT AND CEO, FEDERAL RESERVE BANK OF DALLAS, AND SCOTT'S DAD

Since becoming Scott's client, I've lost weight, increased strength and cardiovascular fitness, and have decreased stress levels. Scott is a great motivator who strives to understand his client's lifestyle and fitness needs and works with them to develop a program geared towards their goals.
- **JAN DALEY,** SOFTWARE DEVELOPER AND DOG AGILITY ENTHUSIAST

With Scott's emphasis on total fitness training, I can tell that cross training and resistance training have helped my running, while his flexibility training program has helped prevent injuries and improve my physical alignment. I also realize now that running, as a complete fitness program, was not allowing me to maximize my overall fitness level and shape my body.

- **SHEILA CHENG,** SOFTWARE DEVELOPER & 6-TIME MARATHONER, INCLUDING TWO BOSTON MARATHONS

For me, working with Scott is more than just lifting weights, doing agility training or running hills. He's customized his YBYL program so that it's specific to reaching my goals on the tennis court and keeps those goals at the forefront of our training. His attention to detail, positive encouragement and motivation is helping both my mind and body get stronger. I know that with Scott's coaching off the court, I will achieve more on the court! Thanks for your help, Scott.

- **ELIZABETH SCHMIDT,** PROFESSIONAL TENNIS PLAYER

Scott has customized eating and exercise programs for me that have really helped me as a sprinter. I've become stronger and more competitive athletically and have also developed new, healthy habits to guide me throughout my life. Thanks!

- **KRISTI TONN,** DUKE TRACK ATHLETE

In a world where our bodies are not redeemed, we need all the help we can get physically. As the Bible points the way to real spiritual truth, Scott's program points the way to physical overcoming.

- **DR. LANCE WATSON,** PASTOR, HIGH POINTE CHURCH

Your body is the only thing you are guaranteed to keep for a lifetime. It forms the foundation of your earthly existence. Energizing your body enriches your life by enhancing every human capacity. If you lack vitality, nothing else really matters; if you have your health, anything is possible.

— Dan Millman, Everyday Enlightenment

www.ybyl.com

Foreword

Scott McTeer and I were friends at Duke University in the late 1980s. I played basketball and he played tennis—number two singles and number one doubles. We shared a house for a time with two other student-athletes. Scott began a pro tennis career when he graduated in 1988. He returned to Durham a couple of years later to coach tennis players. I was in law school at Duke at the time.

Scott moved to Tampa, Florida, in 1992 to become Director of Tennis at Loehr-Groppel-Etcheberry Sport Science. He then went on to coach pro tennis players for several years before committing his professional life to fitness and nutrition in 1996.

I had become assistant Duke Basketball coach under Coach Krzyzewski, and in 1998 we brought Scott to Duke to work with our players on fitness and nutrition. We were especially concerned about our star sophomore, Elton Brand, who had arrived 25 pounds overweight. Coach K and I had Scott evaluate the team's fitness and nutrition needs. He implemented his recommendation in a series of six more visits to Duke that season. The other coaches and I participated in Scott's program along with the players. To make a long story short, Duke was ranked #1 much of that season and finished ranked number 1 in the end-of-season rankings and Elton appeared on the cover of Sports Illustrated as the consensus National Player of the Year.

I moved on to Missouri as head coach in 1999, but Scott continued his consulting relationship with Duke for two more years. He helped Carlos Boozer in 2001 in much the same way he had helped Elton Brand the first year. Duke won the NCAA championship in 2001.

Ironically, in my first year at Missouri, my star freshman, Arthur Johnson, arrived weighing 295 pounds. I called on Scott to do for Arthur and the Missouri program what he had done earlier for Elton Brand and Duke. Arthur was named Conference Freshman of the Year. Missouri hasn't won the national championship yet, but don't count us out.

When Scott told me he was writing a book on fitness and nutrition I wanted to give it a plug. I've seen the results of his programs, and what he has done for elite athletes he can do for you and me. Your first step to better health and fitness is to buy this book and apply its fundamentals.

- **QUIN SNYDER,**
 UNIVERSITY OF MISSOURI
 MEN'S HEAD BASKETBALL COACH

Table of Contents

Introduction XV
My Story XVI
The Softening of the American Body XIX

1. YBYL - PREPARING FOR SUCCESS 1
   YBYL Seven Step Goal Setting 2
   Measuring Your Progress 5
   YBYL Action Plan and Success Disciplines 7

2. YBYL - EATING PLAN 15
   Overview 16
   The Five YBYL Eating Fundamentals 17
   Periodic Detoxification 33
   YBYL Top Five Nutritional Supplements 34

3. YBYL - FITNESS PLAN 35
   Overview 36
   YBYL Seven Challenges to Your Fitness Success ... 37
   The Five YBYL Fitness Training Fundamentals 39
   YBYL Cardiovascular Fitness 43
   The Three YBYL Fundamentals
      of Cardiovascular Training 45
   YBYL Flexibility Training 47
   The Three YBYL Fundamentals of Flexibility Training .. 48
   YBYL Resistance Training 50
   The Three YBYL Fundamentals of Resistance Training .. 51

4. YBYL - WORKBOOK 57
   Overview 58
   Section 1: Preparing for Success 59
   Section 2: YBYL Eating Plan 64
   Section 3: YBYL Fitness Plan 68
   Action Items and Critical Success Factors 70

5. YBYL APPENDIX 71
- YBYL Sample Weekly Training Log 72
- YBYL 28-Day Jumpstart 74
- YBYL Program Summary 82
- YBYL Weekly Training Log 84
- YBYL Food Pyramid 88
- YBYL Two-Day De-Tox Eating Plan 90
- YBYL Super Foods List 91
- YBYL Super Foods Grocery List 95

YBYL Daily Eating Plan (40% protein, 30% carb, 30% fat)
Daily Calories / Daily Amounts **98**
- 1200 Calories, Meal and Snack Plan 100
- 1500 Calories, Meal and Snack Plan 101
- 1800 Calories, Meal and Snack Plan 102
- 2100 Calories, Meal and Snack Plan 103

YBYL Daily Eating Plan (40% protein, 40% carb, 20% fat)
Daily Calories / Daily Amounts **104**
- 1200 Calories, Meal and Snack Plan 106
- 1500 Calories, Meal and Snack Plan 107
- 1800 Calories, Meal and Snack Plan 108
- 2100 Calories, Meal and Snack Plan 109

YBYL Daily Eating Plan (30% protein, 50% carb, 20% fat)
Daily Calories / Daily Amounts **110**
- 1200 Calories, Meal and Snack Plan 112
- 1500 Calories, Meal and Snack Plan 113
- 1800 Calories, Meal and Snack Plan 114
- 2100 Calories, Meal and Snack Plan 115

YBYL Sample Fitness Programs **117**

YBYL Sample Cardio-Muscular Training Workouts **123**

YBYL Super Stretches **127**

YBYl Sample Resistance Training Programs **133**

YBYL Resistance Training **136**

YBYL Resistance Training Form - Upper Body **156**

YBYL Resistance Training Form - Lower Body **157**

I beseech you bretheren, by the mercies of God, that you present your bodies a living sacrifice, holy, acceptable to God, which is your reasonable service.

— Romans 12:1

Introduction

I'd like to offer my congratulations that you're reading these words, because it means that you're more than just a little bit interested in shaping your body, looking younger, feeling and performing better and living longer. You've taken a big step in the right direction. Where you go from here is up to you. However, I want you to know that I'll do everything I can to positively influence and urge you along this path. When I say that I'm 100 percent committed to helping you set and achieve your goals, I truly mean it. Coaching and training people is my mission and I truly love what I do.

Although I could have written a thick book that covers the vast subjects of nutrition and fitness, doing so would have been a disservice to both of us. There are thousands of books on these subjects, most of which do a good job providing you with more information. My goal was to write a "lean" book that provides you with the fundamentals – the tried-and-true techniques and knowledge that you can use to get the results you want.

I should also tell you that 15 percent of my clients don't change their firmly entrenched habits and behaviors. It's easy to quit and give up. However, 85 percent of my clients have achieved substantial results. I challenge you to become a success story by committing to the Your Body, Your Life program and getting a friend or family member to join you.

What excites me about my life is striving to improve in all areas – physically, mentally, emotionally and spiritually. Although Your Body, Your Life focuses on positive physical transformation, I'm equally committed to positive mental, emotional and spiritual transformation, and believe that improvements in all areas will translate into a better, more purposeful life.

Understanding that these pursuits are a lifelong endeavor, I feel blessed to be able to help others along this grand path. Through teaching and coaching, I continue to learn, grow and know. I thank you for this opportunity and wish you the best on your journey.

Because most of this book was written prior to my commitment to God in February 2003, I want to emphasize that God can be your greatest source of strength as you strive to achieve your health and fitness goals! Daily prayer can be our #1 success discipline. God wants to help you have great physical health, and I do too! God Bless You!

- **SCOTT McTEER, CSCS, CPT**
  AUSTIN, TEXAS

My Story

In 1982, I was 18 and was the Maryland high school tennis champion. I'd won the 18-and-under mid-Atlantic championships (Maryland, Virginia and D.C.). I weighed 170 pounds and had seven percent body fat. In 1989, I was 25 and a professional tennis player. I weighed 183 pounds and had seven percent body fat. In 1993, I was 29 and the tennis director for a major sport science firm. I weighed 190 pounds and had 12 percent body fat.

And, in 1995, I was 31 and the national merchandising manager for a publishing company. I weighed 200 pounds and had 19 percent body fat. In this job for a company that was doing $70 million in annual revenue, I oversaw four regional managers, 25 Territory Managers, and more than 300 part-time merchandisers. The demands were high, the stress was real and performance on demand was a job requirement. During that time, I neglected my health, developed horrible eating habits, and didn't exercise regularly. I also put on 10 pounds of body fat and lost several pounds of muscle in one year!

Ultimately, I burned out professionally and realized I was heading down the wrong path. What I didn't know then that I realize now is that performance and happiness vitally depend on taking care of yourself physically. It's your body – it's your life. Had I stayed on my sedentary path of 1995 and not done anything substantial to interrupt my own physical demise, I probably would have lost a pound of muscle and added three pounds of body fat per year.

HOW MY BODY MIGHT HAVE TURNED OUT:

- 1997: 204 pounds and 21.5 percent body fat
- 1999: 208 pounds and 24 percent body fat
- 2001: 212 pounds and 27 percent body fat

Had I not done anything, the numbers would have risen twice as fast! Fortunately, in 1997, I recognized that I was destroying myself physically – and was less than fully satisfied professionally. I decided to return to coaching professional tennis players. It was then that I began to consider becoming a personal fitness trainer. When a player's father died suddenly of a massive heart attack at the age of 55, my destiny was sealed. In 1999, I started a personal fitness training company and became totally committed to helping people reclaim their bodies and live longer, higher quality lives. The changes in my own life inspired me to pursue my new-found professional passion – eating and exercise – as well as get my body back into shape.

HOW MY BODY ACTUALLY TURNED OUT:

- 1997: I weighed 185 pounds and had 18 percent body fat.
- 1999: I weighed 172 pounds and had 7 percent body fat.
- 2002: I weighed 188 pounds and had 7 percent body fat.

But this book and program isn't about me. It's about you. Chances are, most of you can relate to my experience. When we're young, we're more active, exercise regularly, and food is fuel. As we get older, we age gracefully only to the extent that we continue to be active, continue to exercise regularly and continue to view food primarily as fuel. If we don't, our bodies will burn unused muscle as fuel and store lots of body fat.

I'm here to help you reclaim your body – to make sure that you age gracefully and look younger than your years. And to help you feel and perform better and live a long, active life. I believe there's an athletic body in each of us – ready to be built and refined. I believe that we're all athletes – athletes for life. And you don't need to change your career path to achieve dramatic positive changes in your physical well-being. This program is simple, logical and do-able for people of all ages. And, it's one you can use throughout your life. If you're ready to begin, I'm ready to be your coach.

WE CAN GET THERE TOGETHER!

I can't get you to Dallas in 15 minutes and I can't drive you; you have to drive yourself. But I can tell you how to get there. Although some maps are better than others and some won't even get you where you want to go, the truth is that even with the best map, you still have to do quite a bit of driving. The road is somewhat treacherous and there are many ways to go astray. However, you can do it if you really want to. So, I invite you to get fired up and enjoy the ride, even if it means you'll have to make some substantial changes. If you stick with me, it may just be one of the best rides of your life!

— *Scott*

*Knowing is not enough; we must apply.
Willing is not enough; we must do.*

— Johanne von Goethe

www.ybyl.com

The Softening of the American Body

I truly believe that the best way to motivate others is through positive reinforcement. Yet I also believe that when major changes are necessary – when our entire paradigms must shift – it's best to focus on the pain of not changing, in addition to the benefits of doing so. After all, we're motivated to seek pleasure and to avoid pain. My intention is to motivate you to embrace eating and exercise so that you will feel and perform better, look younger, shape your body and live longer.

From my vantage point, Americans are becoming softer and weaker every month – and the momentum is going the wrong way. Anyone who has studied the statistics on adult and adolescent obesity would agree we have a crisis on our hands that's going to keep a lot of doctors busy and make a lot of people unhappy. We simply must adopt more of a preventive approach and truly embrace the role of great fitness and nutrition habits.

As a passionate, results-driven fitness and nutrition coach, I want to solve this crisis through education, information, motivation, the desire for "big carrots" (shaping your body, looking younger, feeling and performing better, and living longer) and the fear of "big sticks" (Type 2 diabetes, cardiovascular disease, cancer, and other diseases). I want to help coach us back to the time when mental and physical fitness was highly valued – even revered. In some ways, I'm a fitness and nutrition evangelist; I'm passionate about my beliefs. Perhaps this is because I've been "born again" with regard to eating nutritiously and exercising regularly. I was on another road, heading down the wrong path. I ate poorly, didn't exercise and let my body go. But, I believe my message is a good one. I hope you'll agree.

Two roads diverged in a wood, and I, I took the one less traveled by, and that has made all the difference.

— Robert Frost, The Road Not Taken

ACCORDING TO *THE U.S. SURGEON GENERAL'S CALL TO ACTION TO PREVENT AND DECREASE OVERWEIGHT AND OBESITY* ISSUED IN DECEMBER 2001:

- 61% of adults in the United States were overweight or obese in 1999. Obesity among adults has doubled since 1980.

- 13% of children and adolescents were overweight in 1999. Obesity among children and adolescents has tripled since 1980.
- 300,000 deaths each year in the United States are associated with obesity.
- Overweight and obesity are associated with heart disease, certain types of cancer, type 2 diabetes, stroke, arthritis, breathing problems, and psychological disorders, such as depression.
- The total direct and indirect costs attributed to overweight and obesity amounted to $117 billion in 2000.
- Studies show that even moderate weight excess (10 to 20 pounds for a person of average height) increases the risk of death, particularly among adults aged 30 to 64 years. Obese individuals have a 50 to 100% increased risk of premature death from all causes, compared to individuals with a healthy weight.
- Less than 33% of Americans meet the federal recommendations to engage in at least 30 minutes of moderate physical activity at least five days a week, while 40 percent of adults engage in no leisure-time physical activity at all.
- High blood pressure is twice as common in adults who are obese than in those who are at a healthy weight.
- More than 80% of people with diabetes are overweight or obese.
- Overweight and obesity are associated with an increased risk for some types of cancer including endometrial (cancer of the lining of the uterus), colon, gall bladder, prostate, kidney, and postmenopausal breast cancer.
- Obesity is associated with a higher prevalence of asthma and sleep apnea (interrupted breathing while sleeping).
- For every 2-pound increase in weight, the risk of developing arthritis is increased by 9 to 13%. Symptoms of arthritis can improve with weight loss.
- Type 2 diabetes, previously considered an adult disease, has increased dramatically in children and adolescents. Overweight and obesity are closely linked to type 2 diabetes.
- Overweight adolescents have a 70% chance of becoming overweight or obese adults.

The fact is, our society is facing many challenges. Whether it's diet, exercise or disease, we could be doing a lot better. Here are some examples:

- **DIET / NUTRITION**
  Consider that people are carrying too much body fat. Too many people have gotten lazy, lethargic and sluggish. Too many people are dehydrated, indirectly resulting in a slower metabolism and excess body fat. We consume too much sodium, indirectly resulting in a slower metabolism and excess body fat. Too many people have the wrong mindset when it comes to fitness and nutrition. Too many people are tired and have a hard time focusing because of what and how they eat.

Too many people haven't heard of the Glycemic Index. Too many people have given up on eating nutritiously and exercising regularly, and have become gluttons for the instant buzz that many non-nutritious foods provide. Even schools are doing a poor job feeding our children.

Too many people don't want to make the connection between what, when and how often they eat, and how they feel. The fact is, too many people are cranky and in bad moods because of what and how they eat. Too many corporate offices have bottomless bowls of candy and cookies and not enough bowls of apples and fresh strawberries. Too many people don't understand how their metabolism works. Too many people skip meals and then overeat later.

We are also drinking refined fruit juices, not realizing we are actually drinking sugared water that is fortified with trace amounts of vitamins and minerals. And too many adults and children are drinking sodas made with refined sugar. And when it comes to diets, there's more starch, sugar and sodium in the American diet than ever. And most doctors are too far from the cutting edge of nutritional science. Even lots of personal trainers aren't always in great shape and don't eat very nutritiously.

- **EXERCISE**

People also equate taking care of their bodies and yes, even shaping them, with being vain - rather than with maintaining good health. We spend too much time finding a parking space as close as possible and not enough time walking the extra hundred yards. Too many people are letting grocery stores "give them a hand" with their groceries. Too many people watch sports on television and too few people play them. Too many people think they know what to do for fitness and exercise, when they really don't and try to do it alone when they shouldn't. Too many people are using the escalators in airports. Too many people aren't doing resistance training, though it's vital to maintain muscle mass and bone density as we get older.

- **DISEASE**

Medical costs in this country are at an all-time high. Too many men develop prostate cancer unnecessarily. Too many mothers, fathers, grandfathers and grandmothers are dying too soon. Not enough time and money are spent on preventing disease. Too many people are taking too many prescription medications. Too many people are deficient in critical vitamins and minerals. Too many women get osteoporosis, and too many people get arthritis – when it could have been prevented.

Our culture must change. We must make eating nutritiously and exercising regularly a top priority – if not for ourselves then for our friends and family who want to see us lead long, healthy lives.

If one advances confidently in the direction of his dreams, and endeavors to live the life he has imagined, he will meet with a success unexpected in common hours.

— Henry David Thoreau

www.ybyl.com

YBYL™ Section 1: Preparing for Success

SECTION 1: PREPARING FOR SUCCESS

Your Body, Your Life™

YBYL Seven Step Goal Setting

Setting specific, clear, challenging goals, reviewing them regularly, and building action plans to achieve them, will boost your chance of success. When you have goals that you're working toward daily – posted where you can see them – you tend to make better decisions and take more positive actions.

While it's been estimated that only five percent of Americans have written goals, this five percent are invariably the most successful. If you're unwilling to do this goal-setting exercise as part of the YBYL plan, there's a very good chance you will fail. If you follow these steps, I can almost guarantee your success.

It's no surprise that personal development guru Stephen Covey chose as one of seven habits to "begin with the end in mind." In the YBYL program, your focus is on goals directly related to your body and to your performance. Because this system works equally well for other areas of your life, I strongly encourage you to apply it there, too. Setting clear, specific goals and developing action plans is a skill and a discipline; the more you do it, the better you'll get. Time to get started!

1. **SET CLEAR, EXCITING, MEASURABLE GOALS, PUT THEM IN WRITING, AND DECIDE WHEN YOU'LL ACHIEVE THEM.**

    What do you want and when do you want it to happen? Do you want to lose 10 pounds of body fat? Get stronger or increase bone strength? Look great in a bathing suit? Would you like to have more energy and be more effective in your personal and business life? Would you like to take control over food and exercise and supercharge your body and life? Put your goals in writing and measure your success!

2. **UNDERSTAND WHY YOU WANT TO ACHIEVE YOUR GOALS. CLARITY BEGETS POWER AND ACTION.**

    Once you know what you want, you can move toward getting it. For anyone pursuing a goal, desire and motivation are the number one determinants of success. Bottom line? You've got to want it! On a scale of 1 to 10, your desire should stay consistently in the 8 to 10 range. Stay aware of your motivational level, as it will wane from day to day and even within a day. Realize that it's your job to stay motivated!

3. **COMMIT FULLY TO YOUR GOALS, AND BELIEVE THAT YOU WILL ACHIEVE THEM.**

    Your level of personal commitment will be challenged every day, so accept the fact that you must stay disciplined and focused. You'll have to make some tough choices and replace old habits with new ones. There will be temporary setbacks, tough days, and

SECTION 1: PREPARING FOR SUCCESS

bumps in the road, but you must remain steadfast in your commitment. Decide that you will be successful and accept no other possibility. Again, you've got to believe in yourself and your success!

4. **DEVELOP A COMPREHENSIVE WRITTEN ACTION PLAN.**

   In the absence of daily action, goals are mere fantasies. Because taking consistent action is not easy and at the same time is the foundation of your success, I've included a customizable YBYL Workbook. It will guide you through this process in a simple step-by-step format, but it's up to you to take action!

5. **TAKE ACTION EVERY DAY TOWARD YOUR GOALS.**

   Don't delay, and don't rationalize giving up or not following through. Instead, master the art of taking baby steps. Don't think of your plan as something you have to do; think of it as something you choose to do. Ten minutes of daily exercise is infinitely better than nothing because it means you've at least exercised your take-action muscles. You don't have to be perfect; you just have to be good and commit to getting better!

6. **MEASURE YOUR PROGRESS AND CONTINUALLY IMPROVE YOUR ACTION PLAN.**

   Brian Tracy, my favorite personal development guru, says "What gets measured, gets done." It's true. You must keep score to know how you're doing. Again, consistent progress, not perfection, is the goal. I've included a YBYL Weekly Training Log in the Appendix to help you, and I encourage everyone to take the YBYL 28-Day Jumpstart Challenge. When you first set goals, you may not know exactly how you'll get there. But as you throw yourself into the process, the steps will become clearer, enabling you to build an improved plan. Measure your progress and improve your plan!

7. **CONTINUALLY RE-COMMIT TO YOUR GOALS AND PLAN.**

   Tenacity and commitment are the hallmarks of successful people. Most goals aren't easy to achieve and won't happen overnight. It's easy to stay with your plan when things are going well and you're feeling good. However, your success will largely be determined by what you do when you don't feel like doing it. Trust me on this: If you want to succeed, then renew your commitment on a weekly basis!

It's important that your specific goals be measurable. The benefits listed at the beginning of this book can serve as a fairly comprehensive list of general health goals. I've included a list of specific, measurable goals in the YBYL Workbook that you can choose. You can also add your own specific goals. By completing these exercises, you'll be taking a very important action. You'll write out your top five one-month, three-month and one-year goals. In some cases, your goals and action steps may overlap. As you achieve your goals, you should replace them with new ones, if appropriate, and update your action steps regularly.

SECTION 1: PREPARING FOR SUCCESS

We can rise above our limitations only when we recognize them.

— B.K.S. Iyengar

Measuring Your Progress

WEIGH YOURSELF ON A SCALE.

If you're trying to lose more than five pounds, you should weigh yourself several times each week. In terms of goal-setting, you should weigh at approximately the same time each day (morning is preferable). Do this, and you'll have continual feedback as to how your body reacts to different types and quantities of food and exercise. Rapid initial weight loss is often water loss because of reduced sodium and carbohydrate intake and increased lean protein and fiber consumption. Substantial body weight fluctuations are the result of the same factors. If weighing yourself is stressful, then either re-frame it in your mind or don't weigh yourself. Sharing your weight and weight goals with at least one other person will double your chance of success because you'll have positive accountability!

Here's an example. I conduct 12-week "lean-down" contests with my clients who want to lose body fat. In this contest, everyone knows everyone else's goals and results, so the accountability factor is quite high. In the second week of one contest, eight of the 10 clients who weighed in achieved their goal, losing a combined 14.5 pounds. This wouldn't have happened without clear, specific goals and positive accountability. If you have less than 10 pounds of body fat to lose, go for a goal of a half or three-quarters of a pound weight loss per week. If you have more than 10 pounds to lose, go for three-quarters to one pound per week.

MEASURING BODY FAT.

Although the percentage of fat on your body is probably the best measure of optimum body weight, measuring it is difficult and often very inaccurate, even when done correctly. Options include using skinfold calipers, but they're not always accurate, and they can be uncomfortable. While hydrostatic testing is generally regarded as the most accurate measure, doing so is fairly time-consuming. And unless you're willing to have it done every few weeks, you won't have enough short-term feedback to know how well you're doing with your plan.

While electrical impedance devices are becoming increasingly more accurate in measuring body fat using a low-level electric current, I still believe we're a year or two away from being able to trust their accuracy. Circumference measurements with a tape measure may be effective; however, it's difficult to ensure that these measurements are done in the same way each time.

SECTION 1: PREPARING FOR SUCCESS

CONCLUSION

I encourage my clients to pick an article of clothing that they can't quite fit in comfortably, then try it on as the program progresses. Your body weight, how your clothes fit and visible body fat are the easiest and best indicators of your success. Simply put, the scale and mirror don't lie. And, weighing yourself on a regular basis will give you the best ongoing feedback.

*The achievement of one goal
should be the starting point of another.*

—Alexander Graham Bell

SECTION 1: PREPARING FOR SUCCESS

YBYL Action Plan and Success Disciplines

If you have not already done so, please complete the goal-setting section of the YBYL Workbook. If you have, you should now be very clear about what you want to achieve. If you're not, then spend more time on your goals before going any further. Time and time again, I see clients diving into a workout or eating program before laying the proper mental foundation. This half-hearted effort, although well intended, will most likely fail when not backed up by clear goals that you're truly excited about achieving. Once you've set goals, the YBYL Workbook can serve as your action plan. A YBYL Action Item Form is provided in the Workbook.

SECTION 1: PREPARING FOR SUCCESS

Your Body, Your Life™

YBYL Success Disciplines

The truth is, changing our habits and making real, long-lasting improvements in our lives is difficult. For better or worse, we all have visions of the person that we would like to be. While it's important to love and accept yourself "as is," I'm also a personal development junkie. So, here's a dose of personal development advice.

When making major improvements in your life, there are certain things you can do to increase your chance of success, such as visualization and maintaining a positive mental attitude. Because of my athletic and personal development background, I believe the more you focus on these areas, the greater your chance of success.

When you consistently focus the tremendous power of your mind on clearly defined goals and actions, great things begin to happen. As with most worthy endeavors, when you practice certain success disciplines, you dramatically improve your chance of success. After all, knowing what to do is clearly a prerequisite to success. Equally important, though, is developing the ability to consistently act on what you know. This is particularly true when achieving your goals involves replacing old habits with new ones. Consider the following:

THINK AND TALK POSITIVELY.

If you're successful in other areas of your life, chances are you can also appreciate the tremendous impact of positive thinking. Don't let words like "can't" become part of your vocabulary. If you catch yourself getting discouraged, making excuses or arguing for your own limitations, then snap out of it and give yourself a pep talk - just like a good coach would do. Review your goals and follow your action plan. Be your own success coach and tell yourself that you can and will succeed. The bottom line? Cultivate a winning attitude!

TRANSFORM INEFFECTIVE VALUES AND BELIEFS TO EMPOWERING ONES.

We must first change our values and beliefs to successfully change our behavior. I've included an exercise in the YBYL Workbook to help you do this. For example, if we believe that food is comforting and provides us with instant gratification, then you'll have a difficult time following an eating plan that will achieve your goals. If, on the other hand, you believe that food is fuel for your mind and body and you value having lots of energy, then you'll be more likely to succeed.

IMPLEMENT SUCCESS RITUALS AND ROUTINES.
Great athletes understand the positive impact of rituals on performance. This is because rituals provide powerful, predictable emotional links to behavior. When we mindfully do things in a certain way and in a certain order for a period of time, it becomes easier and more automatic to repeat this behavior.

For example, John's alarm clock goes off at six in the morning during the week. He has trained himself to immediately shut it off and get out of bed. No hesitation. He goes to the kitchen, drinks 12 ounces of water and pours coffee that's been made with the help of an automatic timer into a travel mug. He goes to the bathroom, brushes his teeth and puts on workout clothes, which he's laid out the night before, along with his work clothes.

He kisses his wife goodbye and leaves the house at 6:20 a.m. with his work clothes, coffee and a lunch box that contains a piece of fruit (mid-morning snack), a protein bar (mid-afternoon snack) and an after-workout protein shake that will serve as breakfast. He works out five days a week at the local gym for 45 minutes and is in exceptional shape. He arrives at the office every day at 8:30 a.m. and leaves every day at 5:30 p.m. At 6:00 p.m., every evening during the week, his family has dinner together. Sound too good to be true - or impossible to attain? It's not if you have a plan.

ACCEPT THAT EATING NUTRITIOUSLY AND EXERCISING REGULARLY REQUIRES ORGANIZATION, PLANNING AND SELF-DISCIPLINE.
I often tell my clients that our culture is conspiring against them in terms of eating to achieve their goals. Unhealthful foods are everywhere. And 95 percent of foods in the grocery store should be avoided. Keep foods that aren't good for you out of the house. The bottom line is if it's not there, you can't eat it. This may be the single most important change you adopt from this program. Use the YBYL Grocery List to help you choose what to buy. Make nutritious foods super-convenient. Pack healthful food and carry it with you. And keep bottled water with you all the time.

If you tend to eat poorly when you eat out, then eat out less frequently or have a healthful snack a few hours earlier so you don't arrive famished and over-indulge. When you fail to plan, you plan to fail. Know what you're going to order before you get there; don't be afraid to substitute items and request special orders at restaurants.

SECTION 1: PREPARING FOR SUCCESS

EMBRACE POSITIVE ACCOUNTABILITY.

The more people who know about your goals and your plans for achieving them, the better your chance of success. Sharing this information provides positive accountability and puts your integrity on the line.

MAKE STEADY, GRADUAL IMPROVEMENTS IN YOUR EATING AND EXERCISE HABITS, NOT RADICAL ONES.

A 10 percent improvement in your eating and exercise habits every week for six weeks and another five percent improvement every week for the next six weeks will result in a major, positive life transformation. Focus first on the things you can easily change and get some momentum. Control what you can, while preparing to address more difficult challenges down the road. Focus on what you can do, and begin mentally preparing yourself for the changes ahead. Consistency matters. Embrace some degree of monotony and make your eating and exercise habits a positive, daily ritual. Be gradual, but challenge yourself as well. Don't expect it to be easy.

VIEW FOOD PRIMARILY AS FUEL, NOT AS PLEASURE.

Your metabolism is the physiological process that converts food to energy. A sluggish metabolism means your body isn't burning calories efficiently, and excess calories are stored as body fat. Unless you consciously eat in a way that will restore your metabolism, it will probably remain sluggish. That's why you must view food for what it is - fuel for your body.

If you want to lose fat, you need to speed up your metabolism so your body uses food more efficiently and burns body fat. An analogy I use with my clients is to think of your metabolism as a wood stove. For this stove to operate at peak efficiency, the stove requires the right amount and type of fuel.

As a culture, we've gone overboard in our expectation that food provide us with pleasure and instant gratification. Unfortunately, this view is generally inconsistent with our goals of feeling better, looking better, performing better and living longer. As long as we rate food (and consume it) based on how good it tastes, foods that taste great and aren't good for us in excess will always occupy this exalted place in our minds. Let's face it: at some point, we must make a choice that will make the difference in whether we achieve our goals.

That choice involves retraining ourselves in how we view food. This is not to say that the food you consume consistently will not and should not give you pleasure, but rather that we must redefine how we define pleasure and learn to shop for and

SECTION 1: PREPARING FOR SUCCESS

prepare tasty, nutritious food. Imagine the pleasure of having lots of energy, looking younger than your years, performing at your best, and knowing that you're taking care of your body for the best chance at a long, productive, fulfilling life.

READ – AND THEN WRITE DOWN – POSITIVE AFFIRMATIONS.

Affirmations are strong, positive, personal statements about how you're going to think and act. They serve to override old information and reinforce new, more positive habits of thought and behavior. Affirmations may also be written down or read aloud. Here is a partial list of sample affirmations.

Please choose some of these and add your own in Section 1 of the YBYL Workbook.

SAMPLE AFFIRMATIONS:

- I weigh _____ pounds and feel great. (Write in your goal weight here.)
- Eating healthfully is the rule, not the exception.
- I drink lots of water every day.
- I enjoy nutritious foods.
- I eat five to six small meals per day.
- I never feel either famished or extremely full.
- When I'm going to be away from home or am unable to eat healthfully, I plan ahead and take nutritious foods with me.
- I'm healthy, lean and fit.
- I'm willing and able to pay a price to achieve my goals.
- I love, admire and respect my body.
- Working out and exercising is a fun and vital part of my life.
- I overcome all challenges that come my way.
- I imagine how my success will make me feel.
- I enjoy taking the steps to make my goals a reality.
- I take responsibility for my actions and my successes.

VISUALIZE YOUR SUCCESS.

This technique is one of the most powerful success disciplines I know. As a dedicated athlete, I visualized virtually every day of my life for more than 10 years. If you can see it, you can be it! Constantly seeing mental images of yourself achieving goals helps them become reality. Visualization strengthens your desires and

SECTION 1: PREPARING FOR SUCCESS

beliefs. If you can't close your eyes and see yourself achieving your goals, then you probably won't. If you can and do, you probably will.

DISPLAY INSPIRATIONAL PICTURES.

Although it may seem corny, it works. Inspiring pictures provide positive, powerful emotional links to achieving your goals. Inspirational pictures are powerful, vivid incentives that will help you achieve your goals. Putting your face on a picture of a body that you're working toward and putting it on the refrigerator or next to your desk might seem silly to everyone else, but it will help keep you focused.

CULTIVATE "SUPPORT STAFF": WORKOUT PARTNERS, MENTORS, COACHES, TRAINERS, FAMILY AND FRIENDS.

It's usually a good idea to surround yourself with supportive people when undertaking anything that's challenging. This is true in business, sports, and in eating more nutritiously and exercising regularly. In some cases, you'll want to communicate your goals to the significant people in your life and ask for their support. Maybe you need to find a workout partner or hire a trainer or coach, or have a heart-to-heart talk with your significant other. What about mentors and role models who have habits that you would like to adopt? Tell these people what your goals and plans are, and ask them to hold you accountable. Encourage them to do the same with you. The point it, don't go it alone.

PRAY AND ASK GOD FOR HIS HELP.

START A "SUCCESS JOURNAL."

Many successful people find that writing in a journal helps them stick to their plan. Writing is also a good way to give you a forum for coaching yourself. After all, any action that increases your awareness and strengthens your desire and commitment is worthwhile.

CULTIVATE STRESS-REDUCING ACTIVITIES.

Many people use food to cope with stress. Others go long stretches without eating. But doing either will only add to the problem. It's simple: eating nutritiously and exercising regularly reduces stress. Eating poorly on a regular basis - or not eating at all - brings on additional stress. I truly believe that much of the stress, bad moods and lack of energy and concentration that we experience is a direct result of poor eating habits.

SECTION 1: PREPARING FOR SUCCESS

Pick up any book on behavior modification and you'll probably read about the importance of interrupting the pattern. It's the same with the YBYL plan. Don't try use poor eating habits to cope with stress. Try deep breathing, stretching, a short nap, massage, exercise, positive thinking, inspirational reading, visualization or a short walk. Laugh more; do fun things. Try yoga! Adopting stress-reducing activities will improve your chances of eating better and exercising regularly.

USE YBYL WEEKLY TRAINING LOGS AND COMPLETE THE YBYL 28-DAY JUMPSTART.

What gets measured gets done. Though simplistic, recording your eating and exercise is a very effective way to help keep you on your plan. In the Appendix, I've included a sample YBYL Weekly Training Log to help you measure your progress. For those of you who wish to triple your chance of success, complete the YBYL 28-Day Jumpstart in the Appendix.

DO PERSONAL STRATEGIC PLANNING ON SATURDAY OR SUNDAY.

Review your goals, action plan and your YBYL Workbook. Assess how well you executed your plan that week. Know your action plan for the next week. Plan ahead. Get into the details. Re-commit to your goals and critical success factors. Take action. Visualize your success. Cultivate a positive, goal-oriented attitude. Implement your Success Disciplines.

Set clear, measurable, fitness, nutrition and body-shaping goals and put them in writing. Develop a simple, yet detailed, written action plan that contains all your critical success factors. Embrace and execute the plan. Fall off the plan. Get back on the plan. Revise the plan and update your goals. Repeat this process until you achieve your goals. Then celebrate your successes and set new goals, even if they're maintenance goals.

Please Complete Section 1, Workbook Exercises.

*Healthy self-denial in any form is an act of self-love.
Its purpose is to strengthen our ability to govern our inward urges.*

— Dr. Gerald Mann, Pastor, Riverbend Church, Jesus, B.C.

Section 2: YBYL™ - Eating Plan

SECTION 2: YBYL EATING PLAN

Overview

Although there are thousands of diet and nutrition books on the market today, there's still a lot of confusion about the best way to eat to shape your body, look younger, feel and perform better and live longer. Why is this? My father, an economist and central banker, says that economists agree on 90 percent of economic issues but choose to debate publicly over the other 10 percent, thus giving the false impression that they don't agree on anything. I think the same is true with eating programs. So much time is spent disagreeing on the 10 percent that not enough time is spent conveying the agreement and importance of the 90 percent.

In the interest of marketing and product differentiation, it seems like everyone has a special slant – some unique approach to eating that will strip away body fat. While there have been some breakthroughs in the past 10 years, the fundamentals still apply: body fat comes off slowly and gradually; extreme eating programs rarely last; and moderation and balance are good things. I hope this section clarifies the 90 percent on which we can all agree and makes a big, positive improvement in your life by explaining the fundamentals of healthful eating.

The YBYL Eating Plan will shape your body and help you look younger, live longer and feel and perform better in a safe way. In the interest of simplicity, I will present the science that's involved in accomplishing this only to the extent that understanding it will help you stick to your plan. The American philosopher William James said "The truth is what works." As a personal trainer who has coached more than 75 successful clients, I have a good understanding of what works and what doesn't, and I'd like to share it with you.

SECTION 2: YBYL EATING PLAN

The Five YBYL Eating Fundamentals:

1. Eat the right amount of daily calories that are optimum for achieving your goals.
2. Eat three small or moderate meals and two or three snacks daily.
3. Eat the right amount of protein, carbohydrates and fat that are optimum for achieving your goals.
4. Consume optimum amounts of water, fiber and sodium.
5. Get most of your calories from YBYL Super Foods.

FUNDAMENTAL #1:
EAT THE RIGHT AMOUNT OF DAILY CALORIES THAT ARE OPTIMUM FOR ACHIEVING YOUR GOALS.

Although there's a lot of talk these days about manipulating carbohydrate, protein and fat ratios to lose body fat, the most important factor is how many calories you consume versus how many you burn. Calories consumed beyond those that are used by your body are converted to body fat. Conversely, when your body uses more calories for energy than you consume, body fat is burned as fuel. It's that simple.

But for many people, the thought of "counting calories" has very little appeal. However, because total caloric intake is Eating Fundamental #1, it is important to at least understand this area. If you spend 20 or 30 minutes studying the food count lists I've included in the Appendix, and commit to reading food labels, you'll quickly develop a good sense of how many calories you're consuming. Since a tablespoon of olive oil has more calories than a large bowl of broccoli, relying on food volume can be very misleading and can lead you down the wrong path. By understanding caloric volume, you'll be halfway toward your goals.

To lose one pound of body fat per week, you must burn 3500 calories per week more than you consume - or 500 calories per day.

DETERMINING YOUR OPTIMUM DAILY CALORIC INTAKE

Although this formula doesn't work for everyone because of variations in body composition, daily caloric expenditure and other factors, it's a good starting point for most people.

SECTION 2: YBYL EATING PLAN

Your Body, Your Life™

1. If you want to lose weight, multiply your current weight times 10 to get your daily caloric target.

2. If you want to maintain your weight, multiply your current weight times 15 to get your daily caloric target.

3. To determine the approximate amount of weight you would lose weekly if you followed this plan perfectly, subtract the number in step 1 from the number in step 2. This is your net daily calories burned.

4. Multiply this number by seven to determine net weekly calories burned.

5. Divide this number by 3,500 to determine the number of pounds you would lose per week.

Note: Your YBYL Workbook will guide you through this exercise. Rapid initial weight loss may occur because of decreased carbohydrate and sodium consumption and increased water and fiber consumption.

Strive for excellence, not perfection in your eating habits. When you cheat on your eating plan, enjoy yourself, but exercise damage control and get right back on the plan.

FUNDAMENTAL #2:
EAT THREE SMALL OR MODERATE MEALS AND TWO OR THREE SNACKS DAILY.

You've probably heard this before, and there's a reason: it works. You must eat four to six times each day for your metabolism to burn at optimum efficiency. Going more than four hours without eating usually slows down your metabolism, creates a substantial drop in your blood sugar levels, and makes it difficult to burn body fat and maintain energy stores. When your blood sugar drops too low and you allow yourself to become very hungry, your chances of overeating increase substantially because your survival instinct takes over and supersedes everything else.

Your meals must be relatively small or moderate in caloric size to kick your metabolism into high gear. Eating too many calories will overwhelm your metabolism and make it difficult to burn body fat. That's why it's vital that you understand approximately how many calories you're taking in at any given time. Trust me on this one. Don't skip meals. Plan ahead. Eat light and often. Since digestion is one of the body's most energy consuming processes, when you eat heavy meals or overeat, you slow your metabolism down and the body begins to store fuel as fat. Believe it or not, not eating often decreases the chance that you'll burn body fat. When you don't eat, your brain sends signals to the body to preserve energy and store body fat because it thinks a famine is coming. Your brain will also send signals to consume a lot of calorie-dense foods to prepare.

Once you understand how calorie consumption works, the challenge is to execute it. You must plan ahead and control your environment. Carry the right snacks with you, and plan, organize and practice self-discipline to execute effectively and reach your goals.

NOTE: Studies have consistently shown that much of the weight loss from today's popular diets may come from muscle loss, which will almost inevitably lead to putting even more weight back on the next time around. Why? Because muscle loss reduces your metabolism and your daily caloric requirements. Even when we sleep, our skeletal muscles are responsible for using more than 25 percent of total caloric intake. An increase in muscle increases our metabolism; a decrease in muscle decreases our metabolism. And, when you don't eat regularly, your chances of exercising regularly are greatly compromised.

DETERMINING OPTIMUM MEAL AND SNACK CALORIES

A good starting point is to consume 75 percent of your daily calories as meals and 25 percent as snacks. As an example, let's assume that you weigh 140 pounds and are trying to lose 15. Using the YBYL formula, your optimum daily caloric target is 1,400 calories. You've also decided to eat three small-moderate meals and two snacks spaced fairly evenly throughout the day. With 75 percent of your daily calories consumed as meals and 25 percent consumed as snacks, the breakdown looks like this:

- .75 X daily caloric goal (1400) = Total daily meal calories (1,050)
- Total daily meal calories (1050) / 3 = Optimum meal calories (350)
- .25 X daily caloric goal (1400) = Total daily snack calories (350)
- Total daily snack calories (350) / 2 = Optimum snack   calories (175)

IN SUMMARY:
- Fundamental #1 says that this person should consume 1,400 daily calories
- Fundamental #2 says that the breakdown should look this: breakfast calories (350), mid-morning snack calories (175), lunch calories (350), mid-afternoon snack calories (175), and dinner calories (350)

(Please refer to the Appendix to determine your appropriate calorie amounts.)

SECTION 2: YBYL EATING PLAN

Realistically, you will skip some meals and snacks and overeat others. But don't give up and say it's too difficult. Instead, get back to your plan. Since Eating Fundamental #1 is the most important, if you overeat early in the day, then lower your calorie intake the rest of the day while continuing to eat light and often. If you skip meals or snacks, don't try to consume extra calories later. Committing to these first two Eating Fundamentals will take you a long way towards achieving your goals.

FUNDAMENTAL #3:
EAT THE RIGHT AMOUNT OF PROTEIN, CARBOHYDRATES AND FAT THAT ARE OPTIMUM FOR ACHIEVING YOUR GOALS.

You need three types of macronutrients – protein, carbohydrates and fat – to keep your metabolism burning strong and steady. These nutrients are life-sustaining substances found in foods that work together to supply the body with energy and to regulate growth, and handle maintenance and repair of the body's tissues.

Most people who want to lose body fat get the best results with a ratio that's approximately 30 to 40 percent protein, 20 to 40 percent carbohydrates and 20 to 40 percent fat. If not, the result is usually a compromised metabolism, excess body fat and poor mental and physical performance. In my opinion, extremes on either end won't produce long-term, sustainable results. Here's an overview of these three important nutrients:

PROTEIN:

After water, protein is the second most plentiful substance in our bodies and makes up about one-fifth of our body weight. Muscles, skin, hair, nails, eyes and many hormones and enzymes are mostly protein.

- As an energy source, one gram of protein yields four calories.
- Protein provides amino acids needed to build, repair and maintain all body tissues.
- Protein helps fight infection by forming disease and infection fighting antibodies.
- As an enzyme, protein assists with essential chemical reactions in the body.
- As a hormone, protein helps regulate body functions.
- Protein may be used for energy or converted to body fat.
- Consumption of protein releases glucagons, a fat-burning hormone.
- Individual protein requirements vary according to size and activity level, with more active individuals having higher optimum protein (and caloric) requirements.

CARBOHYDRATES:

Carbohydrates are converted to glucose the body can use for energy. When you wake up in the morning, your blood probably contains between 70 and 120 milliliters of glucose in each 100 milligrams of blood. This is a normal range and is accompanied by a feeling of alertness and well being. If you don't eat, your blood glucose level will gradually fall as your body draws on a diminishing energy supply. At 60 or 65 milligrams per 100 milliliters – the low end of the normal range – you're beginning to get hungry. The normal response is to eat to increase blood glucose levels. It's important, however, to keep your blood glucose level from rising too high, since that's not good for your body, either.

Insulin is the body's mechanism for attacking blood-sugar spikes. Over time, your body's insulin response may work less effectively due to eating too many non-fibrous carbohydrates. As a result, the body produces excess insulin, which diminishes blood sugar levels and can leave you feeling shaky and hungry. This condition is known as hypoglycemia. Ironically, even with this extra insulin, people are often less able to transport energy-sustaining glucose to their muscles. In a vicious cycle, their body produces more insulin so that ultimately they're unable to produce it, and they become diabetic.

Keeping your blood sugar level constant gives your body a chance to heal from the effects of excessive insulin, which include water and sodium retention, arterial plaque formation, high blood pressure, and excess body fat. The key to stable blood sugar is the reduction and moderation of total carbohydrates and the reduction of non-fibrous carbohydrates.

Finally, carbohydrates also have what is known as a "protein sparing" effect. When you eat the right balance of carbs, protein, and fat, the carbohydrates provide enough glucose for the body, eliminating the need to break down and metabolize muscle into glucose. This process preserves lean muscle and maximizes fat burning. When your diet is properly balanced, your hormonal response allows the muscles to access and burn stored body fat for energy, sparing glucose for the brain.

CARBOHYDRATES AND THE GLYCEMIC INDEX

It's important to know that the effect of foods on blood glucose levels depends on many factors. Not all carbs have the same impact on blood glucose. These effects are explained by a system called The Glycemic Index, which rates how fast certain foods increase blood glucose levels and how quickly the body responds by bringing levels back to normal. The index was originally developed for diabetics and all

SECTION 2: YBYL EATING PLAN

foods were compared to pure glucose, which is rated at 100. The higher the glycemic index, the faster it raises blood sugar. The lower the glycemic index, the slower blood sugar will rise. The glycemic index of a food depends on the type of sugar in the carbohydrate, the amount of fiber, and how the food is cooked or processed.

Carbohydrates that quickly empty into the bloodstream (high-glycemic) are best for immediately after exercise, because the raised blood glucose levels facilitate glycogen synthesis (energy stored in the muscles). Other times, we should strive to eat low or medium glycemic carbohydrates. Understanding the Glycemic Index is especially important for diabetics (and to prevent diabetes), but we now know that everyone from athletes and overweight individuals to those who just want to feel better can benefit.

At least 50 percent of your carbohydrate intake should be low to medium glycemic foods – foods that are high-fiber, low-starch and low-sugar.

- As an energy source, one gram of carbohydrates yields four calories.
- Carbohydrates supply energy to the brain, nervous system and muscles and aid in the absorption of other foods.
- Carbohydrates help metabolize fat and form nonessential amino acids.
- In combination with protein, carbohydrates are essential to fighting infection, lubricating the joints and maintaining the health of bones, skin, nails, cartilage and tendons.
- Carbohydrates contain fiber, which helps to efficiently eliminate waste from the body.
- Carbohydrates that aren't used immediately by the body for energy are either stored as body fat or stored in the muscles or liver as glycogen. If the body doesn't get enough carbs to supply energy needs, it will burn dietary fat, body fat and protein for energy.

FATS: AT LEAST 50 PERCENT OF YOUR FAT INTAKE SHOULD BE UNSATURATED.

- As an energy source, one gram of fat yields nine calories.
- Fat is a nutrient that is often misunderstood, but fulfills unique body functions.
- Fat provides a concentrated energy source.
- Fat is a source of linoleic acid – an essential hormone-building nutrient the body can't make on its own.
- Fat aids in the absorption of fat-soluble vitamins such as Vitamins A, D, E and K.
- Fat carries the flavor of foods.

SECTION 2: YBYL EATING PLAN

- Fat helps maintain body temperature.
- Fat forms structural and functional components of cell membranes and facilitates the digestion and metabolism of other nutrients.
- Fat comes in saturated form (solid at room temperature), trans-fatty acids (semi-solid at room temperature) and in unsaturated form (liquid at room temperature). Unsaturated fats come in either polyunsaturated form (good) or monounsaturated form (best).
- Monounsaturated fats lower your bad cholesterol (HDL) and raise your good cholesterol (LDL).
- Polyunsaturated fats lower your bad cholesterol and raise your good cholesterol.
- Saturated fats raise your bad cholesterol and raise your good cholesterol.
- Trans-fatty acids raise your bad cholesterol and lower your good cholesterol.

In contrast to many popular diets that I believe are too low or too high in any one macronutrient (protein, carbohydrates or fat, for example), I like for people to follow a ratio of macronutrients that will release powerful fat-burning hormones (glucagon) and inhibit the release of fat-storing hormones (insulin). Eating this way keeps your blood sugar balanced and allows your metabolism to burn at a strong, steady rate throughout the day. Dietary fat, protein and fiber all slow down the absorption rate of carbohydrates, providing a time-released supply of glucose. This keeps the fat-storage hormone insulin low. By ensuring that you are consuming carbs that are predominantly high in fiber and low in starch and sugar, the body is able to keep fat-storing insulin at low levels.

IN A NUTSHELL, HIGH-CARB DIETS (LOW FAT, LOW PROTEIN):

- May cause hyperglycemia (high blood sugar) followed by hypoglycemia (low blood sugar).
- May stimulate the release of the fat storage hormone insulin.
- May prevent fat burning by slowing down your metabolism.
- May create cravings for carbohydrates and other foods.
- May lead to mood swings, poor mental focus and lack of concentration.
- May lead to muscle loss and water retention.

HOWEVER, THE OTHER EXTREME OF THE SPECTRUM HAS ITS OWN PROBLEMS, TOO. IN A NUTSHELL, PROLONGED LOW-CARB DIETS (HIGH PROTEIN/HIGH FAT):

- May create hypoglycemia (low blood sugar).
- May slow down your metabolism.

SECTION 2: YBYL EATING PLAN

- May lead to muscle loss.
- May lead to low energy, lack of mental focus and mood swings.
- May lead to rapid weight gain when your brain demands carbs.
- May lead to ineffective fitness workouts.

Most of these diet plans are a continuous subject of debate among the nutritional community. In any event, I believe it's a big mistake if you don't know what nutrients are in the foods you eat. Accept the fact that there's an optimum protein-carb-fat ratio that works best for you. Also accept that this ratio may have to be more aggressive (less starch/sugar/carbs, for example) while you're trying to lose weight than it will be once you've achieved your goal.

DETERMINING YOUR OPTIMUM PROTEIN-CARBOHYDRATE-FAT AMOUNTS

40% PROTEIN / 30% CARBOHYDRATES / 30% FAT WORKS WELL IF YOU ARE:

- Trying to lose weight
- Sensitive to carbs (they create a substantial rise in blood sugar)
- Already used to limiting your carb intake
- Fairly active and work out with medium intensity two to five days per week
- Want to reduce water retention by reducing carb consumption

If you use this eating plan, at least 50 percent of your carbs should be low/medium glycemic (non-sugar/non-starch), and at least 50 percent of your fat consumption should be unsaturated.

40% PROTEIN / 40% CARBOHYDRATES / 20% FAT WORKS WELL IF YOU ARE:

- Trying to lose weight
- Not very sensitive to carbs (they don't create a substantial rise in blood sugar)
- Already used to watching your fat intake
- Working out with medium/high intensity four to six days per week

With this eating plan, at least 50 percent of your carbs should be low/medium glycemic (non-sugar/non-starch), and at least 50 percent of your fat consumption should be unsaturated.

30% PROTEIN / 50% CARBOHYDRATES / 20% FAT WORKS WELL IF YOU ARE:

- Trying to maintain your current weight
- Not sensitive to carbs (they don't create a substantial rise in blood sugar)

SECTION 2: YBYL EATING PLAN

- A vegetarian
- Working out with high intensity four to six days per week or are a competitive athlete

With this eating plan, at least 50 percent of your carbs should be low/medium glycemic (non-sugar/non-starch), and at least 50 percent of your fat consumption should be unsaturated.

Since this is just a starting point and no two individuals are alike in their caloric needs, you should adjust the amount of calories from fat versus carbs, based on how much energy you have and the results you're getting. It has been my experience that many people place too much emphasis on how much carbs versus fat versus protein they're eating – and not enough focus on how many calories they're taking in and how many meals and snacks they're eating. Many people also focus too much on how many carbs they're consuming and too little on the quality of the carbs (sugar, starch, fibrous, etc.), so be careful not to make those mistakes.

Optimum Protein-Carbohydrate-Fat Meal and Snack Amounts

Since there are four calories per gram of protein and carbohydrate and nine calories per gram of fat, the optimum protein-carb-fat amounts would look like this:

40% PROTEIN / 40% CARBOHYDRATES / 20% FAT
1400 daily calories

- 560 protein calories (140g)
- 560 carb calories (140g)
- 280 fat calories (31g)

350 meal calories (breakfast/lunch/dinner)

- 140 protein calories (35g)
- 140 carb calories (35g)
- 70 fat calories (8g)

175 snack calories (mid-morning and mid-afternoon)

- 70 protein calories (18g)
- 70 carb calories (18g)
- 35 fat calories (4g)

SECTION 2: YBYL EATING PLAN

40%-PROTEIN / 30%-CARBOHYDRATES / 30%-FAT

1400 daily calories
- 560 protein calories (140g)
- 420 carb calories (105g)
- 420 fat calories (47g)

350 meal calories (breakfast/lunch/dinner)
- 140 protein calories (35g)
- 105 carb calories (26g)
- 105 fat calories (12g)

175 Snack Calories (mid-morning and mid-afternoon)
- 70 protein calories (18g)
- 53 carb calories (13g)
- 53 fat calories (6g)

30%-PROTEIN / 50%-CARBOHYDRATES / 20%-FAT

1400 daily calories
- 420 protein calories (105g)
- 700 carb calories (175g)
- 280 fat calories (31g)

350 meal calories (breakfast/lunch/dinner)
- 105 protein calories (26g)
- 175 carb calories (44g)
- 70 fat calories (8g)

175 snack calories (mid-morning and mid-afternoon)
- 53 protein calories (13g)
- 88 carb calories (22g)
- 35 fat calories (4g)

If this seems complex, don't worry. Your YBYL Workbook and Appendix will help guide you to your optimum plan. As you get further into the program, understanding and determining caloric volume and protein, carbohydrate and fat breakdowns will become second nature.

SECTION 2: YBYL EATING PLAN

THE 80/20 RULE FOR LOSING BODY FAT

If your goal is to lose body fat, 80 percent of your results will be the result of your eating habits. While great eating habits can make up for poor exercise habits, great exercise habits can't make up for poor eating habits. Put another way, 30 seconds of poor eating can easily erase 30 minutes of great exercise. Pay attention to the quantity and quality of food you're eating, and make conscious, intelligent decisions based on your goals.

FUNDAMENTAL #4:
CONSUME OPTIMUM AMOUNTS OF WATER, FIBER AND SODIUM.

WATER

Water is truly nature's gift to power performance and also a potent, indirect way to burn fat. Since just about every cell of your body needs water to function at peak levels, denying your body its water needs will indirectly slow down your metabolism and encourage your body to store fat. Water helps remove waste products from the kidneys, detoxifies the liver, improves skin tone, helps metabolize fat and flushes out toxins from your body. If you're concerned about retaining water, here's a paradoxical truism: Drink water to lose excess water. It really works!

Water is also necessary to allow for regular easy elimination. If we don't drink enough water, the mucous lining of the colon becomes hard and fails to provide a slick surface for waste to move out of the body. Water is fiber's best friend!

Recommendation: Drink water all day, starting with 12 to 16 ounces first thing in the morning. Drink at least three-quarters of an ounce of water for every pound of body weight daily. For example, for a 140-pound person, you'd need to drink at least 105 ounces a day.

FIBER

Fiber is a type of carbohydrate chain that can't be broken by the body and that is too large to be absorbed though the intestinal wall and pass through the digestive tract unbroken. Fiber comes in two forms: soluble (dissolves in water) and insoluble (doesn't dissolve in water). Soluble fiber slows the absorption rate of sugar into the bloodstream and lowers blood cholesterol levels. Insoluble fiber also slows down the absorption of sugar into the bloodstream and speeds up the rate that food is passed through the digestive tract.

SECTION 2: YBYL EATING PLAN

A high fiber diet reduces your chance of getting colon or rectal cancer by allowing carcinogens in food to move faster through the intestines. Fiber is also essential for providing bulk to allow for easier elimination of waste through the colon. It also absorbs fats and toxins and helps eliminate them from the body. Think of fiber as the "Liquid Plum'r" of food. Fiber also gives you the sensation of being full and makes it less likely that you'll overeat.

Recommendation: Divide your body weight by six to determine the amount of daily fiber that's optimum for you. Invest in soluble fiber capsules, pure oat or wheat bran, or other soluble fiber supplements like Metamucil - and take them daily. Refer to your YBYL Super Foods List in the Appendix for a list of high fiber foods.

SODIUM

Sodium is an essential mineral because it helps regulate body fluid balance and volume, is necessary for normal muscle tone, nerve function and heart function, and aids in converting glucose to glycogen. Most people require less than 1000 milligrams per day. Athletes and avid exercisers need more, since sodium is also an electrolyte mineral that's eliminated when we sweat.

Most of us don't need to worry about getting enough sodium, however, because the average American consumes 3,000 to 6,000 milligrams of sodium per day – far too much for optimum health. Besides increasing blood pressure to unhealthy levels, excess sodium leads to water retention and bloating.

Reducing sodium intake to healthy levels decreases calcium loss and increases calcium absorption, which may reduce bone demineralization and bone loss. Since most of the sodium in our diet comes from processed foods and table salt, not eating those foods - especially high-sodium canned goods, soups and frozen foods - and avoiding table salt will do wonders. Try a salt substitute or other seasoning, and search for low-sodium foods. Beware of restaurants that load healthful foods with fatty condiments and high-sodium sauces. Read labels and search out low-sodium options for your favorite foods – they're out there. The following is a list of high-sodium foods to avoid:

Recommendation: Unless you have a higher than average need for sodium, limit your intake to 10 milligrams for each pound of body weight.

SECTION 2: YBYL EATING PLAN

High Sodium Foods

FOOD	Sodium (mg)	Calories
Bacon (3 slices)	303	135
Barbeque sauce (1 tablespoon)	156	21
Barbequed beef (1 tablespoon)	84	25
Beef, jerky (1 oz)	627	116
Bologna (1 oz)	295	90
Canadian bacon (3 oz)	1,315	157
Catsup (1 tablespoon)	178	16
Cheese - American (1 oz)	406	106
Cheeseburger, large, 1 patty, (4 oz raw), fully loaded	787	324
Chicken breaded, fried, breast & wing	536	249
Chicken-fried steak, prepared in restaurant, (12 oz)	1,281	1,066
Corned beef (3 oz)	964	213
Cottage cheese - 2% fat (1/2 cup)	459	101
Burrito w/ beans, cheese, beef (2)	875	518
Egg drop soup (1 cup)	1,064	90
Fish sandwich w/ tarter sauce & cheese (1)	1,403	507
Frankfurter (1)	642	102
French fries (4 oz)	224	332
Fried rice (1 cup)	411	223
Luncheon meat, olive loaf (1 oz)	374	76
Macaroni & cheese, w/ whole milk, (1 cup)	1,152	482
Olives, green (10 small)	696	34
Pastrami, beef (1 oz)	380	41
Pepperoni (1 oz)	578	141
Pickle, dill, 3 3/4" long (1)	833	12
Popcorn, "buttered" & salted (6 cups popped)	984	637
Potato chips (1 oz)	183	156
Potato salad, prepared w/ mayo, (1/2 cup)	293	209
Pretzels (1 oz or about 5 pretzels)	486	108
Rice, seasoned mixes, prepared w/ margarine (1 cup)	785	275
Salad dressing, French (1 tablespoon)	190	56
Salami (1 oz)	527	119
Salt (1 teaspoon)	2,358	0
Sausage, pork, smoked	880	251
Soup, chicken noodle, prepared w/ water, (1 cup)	951	76
Soy sauce (1 tablespoon)	911	8
Sweet & sour chicken (2 cups)	3,005	1,183
Tomatoes, canned, stewed (1/2 cup)	347	37
Tuna, canned in oil, drained (3 oz)	301	168
Vegetable juice cocktail (6 fl oz)	490	34
Wonton soup w/4-5 wontons (1 cup)	1001	235

SECTION 2: YBYL EATING PLAN

FUNDAMENTAL #5:
GET MOST OF YOUR CALORIES FROM YBYL SUPER FOODS.

Not all proteins, carbs and fats are created equal. Some foods are burned for energy more efficiently than others and are also better for you. As you've already learned, calories and food combinations are important, as are daily meals and snacks. When you make choices in daily eating, choose from the following list of "super foods" for optimum nutrition:

SUPER FLUIDS:
- Water, green and unsweetened tea, fresh vegetable or fruit juice with no added sugar.

SUPER DIETARY SUPPLEMENTS:
- Soluble fiber capsules, pure oat or wheat bran, sugar-free Metamucil, vitamins in capsule or liquid form.

SUPER SWEETENERS:
- For zero calories, go with Splenda or Stevia and minimize sugar. Fructose is your best sugar and is 50 percent sweeter than sucrose.

SUPER CARBS:
- Grains: breads and cereals that have at least one gram of fiber for every five grams of carbohydrate; high-fiber pasta, oatmeal (slow-cooked).
- Fruits: strawberries, apples, peaches, pears, plums, grapefruit, cherries, berries, oranges, firm bananas, lemons, limes.
- Vegetables: salads, spinach, greens, romaine lettuce, cucumbers, broccoli, celery, cauliflower, cabbage, asparagus, green beans, snow peas, squash, zucchini, sprouts, peppers, onions, mushrooms, radishes, tomatoes. (Raw, steamed or grilled is best; don't overcook or use much salt.)
- Beans, Lentils and Legumes: high-fiber/low-sodium beans and lentils including soy, kidney, black, Great Northern, lima, navy, pinto, garbanzo beans (chickpeas), hummus, black-eyed peas and low-sodium veggie burgers.
- Low-fat Dairy Products: plain/vanilla yogurt, soymilk, low-fat cottage cheese, other low-fat products (assuming no allergies or food sensitivities to dairy).

SUPER FATS:
- Fish, olive, almond and peanut oils, avocadoes, olives, low-sodium nuts and seeds, natural or soy peanut butter (these don't have trans-fatty acids), almond butter and tahini.

SUPER PROTEINS:
- Lean meats, fish, soy products, protein shakes and bars, egg whites, tofu, and low-fat cottage cheese.

THE FOLLOWING FOODS SHOULD BE CONSUMED SPARINGLY:
- Sugar, sugar drinks, refined fruit juices, fruit yogurt, baked beans, ketchup, and sugar products (candy, cookies, cakes, pies)
- Refined junk food (chips, crackers, high-carb "nutrition" bars)
- Low-fiber bread, tortillas, bagels, breakfast cereals, pasta and rice
- Saturated fat and trans-fatty acids
- Fried foods, fatty meats, gravy and other creamy sauces, and full-fat dairy products such as creamy salad dressings, sour cream, solid cheeses and whole-milk cottage cheese
- Excessive sodium and other additives and preservatives, found in frozen, canned or highly processed foods
- Vegetable oils with trans-fatty acids, and other foods that contain trans-fatty acids, such as regular peanut butter
- Diet soft drinks, refined fruit and vegetable juices
- Alcohol, aspartame and saccharin

ALCOHOL:
If you drink, try to limit it to one or two drinks per day. To help flush alcohol toxins from the body, drink an additional 8 to 12 ounces of water for each drink, and take extra antioxidant vitamins (such as vitamins A, C and E, carotenoids and selenium) to offset free radical damage. Free radicals are highly reactive compounds that can cause irreversible damage to body tissues. Free radical damage is also linked to premature aging, cancer, impaired immune function, arteriosclerosis and other disorders. If one of your goals is fat loss, avoid extra calories in your drinks by choosing water and club soda over juices and sugary mixers.

Alcohol-related calories should be factored into your total calories and will influence the rate at which you achieve your goals. Here are calorie counts for some popular drinks.
- One 1.5 ounce shot of 80 proof alcohol has 95 calories
- One 12-ounce light beer has 95 calories
- One 12-ounce regular beer has 150 calories
- One 7-ounce glass of wine has 175 calories

SECTION 2: YBYL EATING PLAN

- One 6-ounce gin and tonic, whiskey and cola, or vodka and cranberry has 165-175 calories
- One 8-ounce margarita with fresh lime juice and 3 ounces of tequila has 310 calories
- One 8-ounce machine-style, pre-mixed margarita with 3 ounces of tequila has 430 calories

Note: If you don't drink, please don't start to drink wine for its antioxidant qualities. For additional antioxidants, supplement with liquid or capsule antioxidant vitamins, use grapeseed extract, and eat more fruits and vegetables. Remember, alcohol is a depressant, decreases your metabolism, increases your need for water and contains a significant amount of calories that have no nutritional value. Too much alcohol can rob your body's ability to absorb other nutrients and is associated with a wide variety of diseases, including cancer and liver complications. Moderate consumption of alcohol will prolong your life and make it easier to achieve your calorie consumption goals.

Please Complete Section 2 Workbook Exercises

Periodic Detoxification

I once read about a natural food expo that featured a Twinkie that was 10 years old and still very much intact. It was so loaded with additives and preservatives that it had easily withstood a decade. In contrast, I drink a protein shake every day mixed with vanilla soymilk and, if I don't rinse out my shaker thoroughly when I'm done, it becomes a stink bomb in less than 24 hours. This is actually a good thing, because it means it's not loaded with the chemicals that keep it from becoming a stink bomb.

Processed foods are loaded with a lot of chemicals and preservatives that permit a long shelf life and make food taste good. However, your body treats these unnatural additives like poison and generally holds onto water in an attempt to flush them out. Because too many additives and preservatives are poisonous to the body, people generally don't feel very good after meals that have them. They may also feel heavier and mistake the extra water for body fat.

The answer is to drink lots of water, particularly if you know you've eaten foods that induce puffiness. If you don't, these additives will just sit there, continuing to poison your body. (Think of the Twinkie!) When you first start drinking water you'll probably feel more bloated, but eventually you'll flush everything out. I don't recommend drinking lots of water before or during a meal because it tends to affect vitamin and mineral absorption.

The good news is if you follow the five YBYL Eating Fundamentals, these bad things are much less likely to happen. But you need to be realistic, too. Let's face it, we can't eat well all of the time. In fact, I encourage my clients to have one or two "reward" meals per week so they can indulge in their favorite foods. But you know that your body – like your house – may need the occasional "spring cleaning" so that you can get rid of waste, toxins and byproducts.

Through periodic detoxification of the body, we can help reduce the amount of toxins that enter the bloodstream. For example, chlorophyll and spirulina drinks are excellent liver cleansing aids and also help to alkalinize blood.

Your immune system's first line of defense is your skin. Toxic build-up and sluggish lymph circulation limits the body's ability to function, as well as causing skin-related health problems such as premature aging of the skin, cellulite and inflammation of the connective tissue, acne breakouts, sensitive, allergic skin, varicose veins; and stretch marks.

SECTION 2: YBYL EATING PLAN

The key to eliminating toxins is to follow your YBYL eating and fitness plan, practice periodic detoxification, do deep breathing and practice yoga, get regular massages, take hot baths with Epsom salts, and use saunas.

The YBYL Top Five Supplements:

1. Water.
2. High-quality multiple vitamin-mineral supplements.
3. Pure wheat bran and soluble fiber supplements.
4. Additional antioxidants (Vitamins A, C, E, selenium, grapeseed extract, green tea)
5. Additional minerals for most adults (calcium, magnesium, zinc, etc.)

WHY YOU SHOULD CONSIDER NUTRITIONAL SUPPLEMENTS

Besides getting regular exercise and eating nutrient-rich foods, you can improve your health, performance, body composition and energy levels by supplementing with vitamins, minerals and digestive enzymes. By facilitating the action of enzymes, vitamins help initiate a wide variety of body responses, including energy production and the growth of healthy tissue. While most nutrition experts agree that food is the single best source of vitamins, minerals and enzymes, surveys often reveal that a large percentage of people don't consume adequate amounts.

In addition, actual absorption of these nutrients may be low, despite getting enough of them through a healthy diet. When your body is deficient in just one essential vitamin or mineral, more than 1,000 chemical and enzymatic processes in your body could be affected. The right amount of micronutrients is crucial to optimum health and performance.

Section 3: YBYL™ Fitness Plan

SECTION 3: YBYL FITNESS PLAN

Overview

Although most adults know they should exercise regularly, most of them don't. Of those adults who do exercise regularly, their program is generally limited and haphazard, rather than comprehensive and progressive. With such a universal acceptance that a regular, comprehensive fitness program is essential to our health and longevity, why is it that more people don't "just do it"?

The important thing is that you are on your way to making a regular, comprehensive fitness program a non-negotiable part of your life. It is important to note, however, that I recommend that you improve your eating habits for a couple of weeks before taking on a new fitness program.

… SECTION 3: YBYL FITNESS PLAN

YBYL Seven Challenges to Your Fitness Success

CHALLENGE #1:
MOST PEOPLE HAVEN'T MADE THEIR FITNESS PROGRAM A PRIORITY AND TRULY COMMITTED TO IT.

Exercise is important, but not urgent. "I'll start next week when I have more time" is something I hear all the time. Until fitness becomes a top priority and you really commit to it, it won't happen. No one else can do it for you. Your commitment level is truly the Number One determinant of your success.

CHALLENGE #2:
MOST PEOPLE ASSOCIATE PAIN AND DISCOMFORT WITH THE IDEA OF WORKING OUT REGULARLY.

No matter how we may sell ourselves on the idea, we still have strong, negative emotional links between displeasure and working out regularly. The solution is to work from the inside out to get rid of those negative associations and replace them with positive ones. For example, as long as you think you don't have time to work out regularly, will you ever have time to work out regularly? No. Mental fitness goes hand in hand with physical fitness.

CHALLENGE #3:
MOST PEOPLE HAVEN'T SET COMPELLING, MEASURABLE FITNESS GOALS AND WRITTEN THEM DOWN.

When goals are unclear, immeasurable and exist only in your head, it's very difficult to get excited about achieving them. What's more, without writing them down and keeping track, we don't even know when we're on course or off.

CHALLENGE #4:
MOST PEOPLE DON'T HAVE AN EFFECTIVE PLAN THAT WILL HELP THEM ACHIEVE THEIR GOALS.

A great plan for success includes action steps, positive accountability, organization and self-discipline. It can't be a whim or a fly-by-the-seat-of-your-pants sort of thing. You have to really get into it! Let me repeat. You have to really get into it! Also, the plan must work. If you're trying to get to Dallas from Austin with a road

SECTION 3: YBYL FITNESS PLAN

map that will take you to Houston, you won't get to Dallas unless you stop and get good directions. And with each successive failed trip, you stop believing that you can get there. The truth is, you need a good road map and you have to get into the trip. And I know how to get there and can give you good directions.

CHALLENGE #5:
MOST PEOPLE TRY TO GO IT ALONE AND DO IT ALL THEMSELVES.

You need a support team. You need to surround yourself with coaches, role models, mentors and people who want you to achieve your goals. Most of us need support, positive accountability and tips to incorporate fitness into our lifestyles.

CHALLENGE #6:
MOST PEOPLE DON'T EAT NUTRITIOUSLY ENOUGH TO HAVE THE ENERGY TO WORK OUT REGULARLY.

As Vince Lombardi once said, "Fatigue makes cowards of us all." It's for this reason that the YBYL Eating Plan was explained before the YBYL Fitness Plan. If you want to succeed with your fitness plan, you must first find success with your eating plan. Each is directly impacted by the other.

CHALLENGE #7:
OUR CULTURE IS CONSPIRING AGAINST YOU.

As the ultimate consumer society, we are conditioned to look for easier, faster ways to do things. Computers are faster and more powerful, the Internet makes us more efficient, medical advances help us live longer, mobile phones are getting better, lawn mowers push themselves, and our remote control television sets provide us with hundreds of choices 24/7/365. While it's a good thing that our standard of living has increased, more adults have become sedentary, even gluttonous and lazy. We get bored easily, can't focus our minds on one thing for very long, and even want to be entertained while we work out. And if we don't feel good, can't concentrate, and are depressed, it's far too easy to visit the doctor and get a pill that will cure our ills, thus ensuring that we're not addressing the source of our angst.

Because of our lifestyles, many adults are waiting for the magic fitness pill or the device that can be worn at night that will get us in tremendous shape in less than three weeks. Stop waiting. Although there are always better ways to do things – and ways to work smarter, not harder – the truth is that substantial, lasting improvements are the result of both hard work and smart work. And the best way to feel and perform better, look younger, shape your body and live longer are the magical elixirs I call nutritious eating and regular exercise.

Your Body, Your Life™ SECTION 3: YBYL FITNESS PLAN

The Five YBYL Fitness Fundamentals:

1. Implement a fitness program that's safe, gradual, progressive, specific and scheduled.
2. Exercise four to five times per week.
3. Follow a customized fitness program that's based on achieving your specific health, fitness, body shaping and sport-specific goals.
4. Implement a well-rounded fitness program that challenges the cardiovascular system, builds muscular strength, endurance & symmetry, and increases flexibility and physical alignment.
5. Implement an efficient fitness program that maximizes results in the time you're investing.

FUNDAMENTAL #1:
IMPLEMENT A FITNESS PROGRAM THAT'S SAFE, GRADUAL, PROGRESSIVE, SPECIFIC AND SCHEDULED.

SAFETY:

If you are about to start a resistance-training program or already doing one, consult a qualified fitness professional to make sure your technique is safe and correct. If you're training with improper form, you'll greatly increase the chance of injury.

WARM UP AND COOL DOWN:

Always warm up before working out. Simply work at a much slower pace in whatever physical activity you've chosen. The purpose of the warm-up is to elevate your body temperature and blood pressure and increase the temperature of muscle and connective tissue, thereby reducing the risk of injury. Warming up also reduces the body's potential for fatigue. Be sure to cool down and stretch after working out to minimize soreness and help with recovery.

GRADUAL AND PROGRESSIVE:

One of the most common mistakes is that people try to do too much too fast. Start slow, be conservative and increase both duration and intensity on a weekly basis. Workouts that aren't gradual and progressive aren't safe. I recommend that those

www.ybyl.com

SECTION 3: YBYL FITNESS PLAN

who are just beginning a regular fitness program spend two weeks on the YBYL Eating Plan first, then add cardiovascular (aerobic) training three to four times per week for a couple of weeks, and then add flexibility training (stretching/yoga) and two to three resistance training or cardio-muscular training sessions per week.

You'll find a progression of ten fitness programs in the Appendix. Refer to this progression and increase your routine every few weeks until you've reached Level 5 or higher. Once you've been training for at least four weeks, train with medium/high intensity and focus on maximizing results versus time invested. Your body doesn't know how many minutes it has been in the gym or how many sets and reps it has done; it only knows how much work it has done and whether it will adapt positively.

BE SPECIFIC AND SCHEDULE YOUR WORKOUTS:

Another common mistake people make is that they're too general about when they'll work out, what they'll do and for how long. Deciding you'll exercise "after work" a few times per week is markedly inferior to deciding you'll work out for 30 minutes at 6 p.m. on Mondays, Tuesdays, Thursdays and Fridays and at 9 a.m. on Saturdays. Deciding that you'll do upper body resistance training on Mondays, lower body resistance training on Thursdays and cardiovascular training on the other days at these specific times is even better. As with goals, specificity helps people become more efficient than when they don't have deadlines. Once you decide exactly when you'll work out and exactly what you'll do and for how long, you're free to organize the rest of your life around these appointments with yourself.

It is never too late to be what you might have been.

— George Eliot

FUNDAMENTAL #2:
EXERCISE FOUR TO FIVE TIMES PER WEEK.

Build up gradually, but start the process. Exercising 15 minutes a day, four times a week is much better than working out 60 minutes a day, once a week. Start with at least three workouts per week and gradually build up to four or five. If you're just starting a program, walking for 15-20 minutes a day is a great way to begin.

SECTION 3: YBYL FITNESS PLAN

Choose specific days and times to do this and put them in your planner, or wherever you'll see it.

Also consider recruiting an exercise partner, training with a group, or hiring a trainer. Studies have shown that beginning exercisers are more successful when they work out with partners or personal trainers. If someone is expecting you to be at a certain place at a certain time to work out, you're more likely to show up. Studies have also shown that people who exercise in groups have twice the commitment of those who try it alone. A partner, training group or personal trainer may help you stay on your program.

TIP: If you work out efficiently, effectively and intelligently, you can have a great fitness program in only 45 minutes a day, five days a week. That's only 3.75 hours a week - just 2.2 percent of your total weekly time. Even if you factor in 15 minutes for commute time, prep, etc., it's still only five hours a week - or 3 percent of your total weekly time. Not working out regularly is rarely a result of not "having time," but almost always a result of not making fitness a priority and developing a plan and the self-discipline to follow through.

FUNDAMENTAL #3:
FOLLOW A CUSTOMIZED FITNESS PROGRAM THAT'S BASED ON ACHIEVING YOUR SPECIFIC HEALTH, FITNESS, BODY SHAPING AND SPORT-SPECIFIC GOALS.

Begin by setting personal, specific and measurable goals and putting them in writing. Make sure these goals are challenging, but realistic. Once you're clear on what your goals are and your specific fitness preferences, you can design a fitness program to achieve them. Of course, achieving your goals will depend greatly on your success in implementing the YBYL Eating Plan and following the Fitness Fundamentals. But don't worry. We've provided all the information you need to help you design and implement a program that's right for you at the end of this section.

FUNDAMENTAL #4:
IMPLEMENT A WELL-ROUNDED FITNESS PROGRAM THAT CHALLENGES THE CARDIOVASCULAR SYSTEM, BUILDS MUSCULAR STRENGTH, ENDURANCE & SYMMETRY, AND INCREASES FLEXIBILITY AND PHYSICAL ALIGNMENT.

The three cornerstones of fitness are cardiovascular endurance, muscular strength and endurance and muscular flexibility. These can be achieved through aerobic training, resistance training and flexibility training. While most forms of aerobic

SECTION 3: YBYL FITNESS PLAN

exercise involve some degree of muscular strength, endurance and flexibility, and most forms of resistance training involve some degree of aerobic and flexibility training, each form is best pursued separately. I also encourage you to do cardio-muscular training-cardiovascular training that significantly challenges the muscular system and shapes the body. Stair-stepping machines or treadmill walking at a high incline are great for this, particularly if you prefer cardiovascular training to resistance training.

> *We are what we repeatedly do.*
> *Excellence, then, is not an act, but a habit.*
>
> — Aristotle

FUNDAMENTAL #5:
IMPLEMENT AN EFFICIENT FITNESS PROGRAM THAT MAXIMIZES RESULTS IN THE TIME YOU'RE INVESTING.

Just as successful people tend to be efficient and effective, the same should hold true with a fitness program. Since your time is limited and precious, training intelligently, effectively and efficiently should be a top priority. Your body does not know how long it was in the gym, however, it does know how much work it did. I would estimate that less than 10 percent of regular exercisers train intelligently, effectively and efficiently. Specific guidelines for efficiency and effectiveness are included later in this section.

TIP:

Many regular exercisers listen to their favorite music on compact disc and tape players. You may want to try this! Or, invest in new workout clothes or buy a new swimsuit to boost your motivation!

YBYL Cardiovascular Fitness

Cardiovascular fitness, also known as aerobic or cardio-respiratory endurance, is the ability of the heart, lungs and blood vessels to deliver adequate oxygen to exercising muscles. Blood must flow from the heart (cardio) through the blood vessels (vascular) to the lungs to pick up oxygen to deliver to exercising muscles. Increasing your aerobic fitness will not only strengthen your heart and lungs, but may also add quality years to your life.

Aerobic means "with oxygen." The aerobic energy system is dominant when enough oxygen is delivered to cells to meet energy needs. Anaerobic means "without oxygen." Without enough oxygen, such as when a muscle needs to generate force quickly, e.g. to lift a heavy weight, the muscle relies primarily on anaerobic systems.

Aerobic exercise is the only physical activity that directly burns body fat. For fat to be burned, oxygen must be present. At the start of aerobic exercise, your body uses carbohydrates - stored as glycogen in the muscles and liver - for energy. After about 20 minutes of working out, fat is released from cells in the form of fatty acids to be used as energy. Although aerobic exercise may burn body fat directly, for most people, the goal should be to burn calories - whether they're carbohydrates in the liver and muscles or body fat. In my opinion, the amount of calories burned during and after exercise is most important.

Aerobic exercise also strengthens your heart muscle, raises the level of (good) high-density lipoprotein (HDL) cholesterol that helps prevent clogged arteries, and lowers your blood pressure, thus reducing your chances of having a heart attack or stroke. There are so many benefits that you should think of aerobic exercise as a lifetime commitment - not something to be done for only a short time.

Optimum exercise intensity for cardiovascular improvement and fat burning is 60 to 85 percent of your maximum heart rate. To determine your maximum heart rate, subtract your age from 220. If you can carry on a comfortable conversation while exercising, then you're probably exercising at a low intensity (50 to 65 percent of your maximum heart rate). If breathing's somewhat labored and difficult, you're probably exercising at a medium intensity (65 to 75 percent). If breathing's difficult, you're probably exercising at a high intensity (75 to 85 percent).

SECTION 3: YBYL FITNESS PLAN *Your Body, Your Life™*

If you're just beginning an exercise program, exercise at low to medium intensity for several weeks, and you'll begin to improve aerobic fitness. If you exercise at a lower intensity, increase the time spent exercising to achieve positive fat-burning and cardiovascular benefits. If you exercise for shorter periods, exercise intensity should be increased so you're getting maximum results.

TYPES OF AEROBIC TRAINING INCLUDE

walking, hiking, jogging, running, elliptical training, cycling, racquetball, handball, squash, jumping rope, tennis, basketball, canoeing, rowing, kayaking, skiing, skating, soccer, rowing, swimming, challenging yoga (such as Ashtanga or Bikram), cross-country skiing, aerobics and stair climbing.

- Aerobic interval training involves periodically increasing and decreasing workout intensity within a workout. This leads to rapid increases in cardiovascular fitness because you're increasing your anaerobic threshold.

    EXAMPLES:
    - Alternately walking for a minute and walking faster or jogging for a minute
    - Alternately jogging for a minute and running faster for 30 seconds
    - Cycling slowly for 30 seconds, then picking up the pace for 30 seconds

- Aerobic cross training involves doing several types of aerobic exercise on a regular basis. Cross training prevents over-use injuries, helps avoid aggravating an existing injury, and allows for greater physical and mental recovery between sessions.

- Cardio-muscular training includes aerobic training that also significantly challenges the muscular system. This type of training is particularly good for people who want to minimize the amount of resistance training they need to do.

- Cardio-muscular training that significantly challenges lower body muscles includes: stair machines, stair climbing, elliptical trainer set on high resistance, cycling, walking on an incline, sprinting or striding (80 percent sprint) on flat ground or uphill, rowing, racquetball, handball, squash, tennis, basketball, kayaking, step aerobics, hiking, skating, blading, snow skiing, water skiing, soccer, challenging yoga and pilates.

- Cardio-muscular training that significantly challenges upper body muscles includes: rowing, racquetball, handball, squash, tennis, kayaking, water skiing, swimming, cycling, elliptical trainers that incorporate arm movements, challenging yoga, cross-country snow skiing and pilates.

The Three YBYL Fundamentals of Cardiovascular Training:

1. Be safe and gradual, yet progressively challenge yourself until you've achieved your desired level of aerobic fitness.
2. Train two to three times per week for at least 30 minutes.
3. Train in a way that maximizes results in the time you're investing.

FUNDAMENTAL #1:
BE SAFE AND GRADUAL, YET PROGRESSIVELY CHALLENGE YOURSELF UNTIL YOU'VE ACHIEVED YOUR DESIRED LEVEL OF AEROBIC FITNESS.

SAFETY.

Develop correct form on all cardiovascular exercises. If you plan on running, make sure you have correct running form. The same is true for all cardiovascular training.

WARM UP AND COOL DOWN.

Always warm up before working out. Cool down and stretch after working out to minimize soreness and facilitate recovery.

GRADUAL AND PROGRESSIVE.

Resist the temptation to do the same workouts at the same intensity for the same duration until you've achieved your aerobic fitness and body shaping goals. Develop the habit of extending your aerobic comfort zone at least every third or fourth workout. If you're bored while you train, then you probably need to increase intensity. Similarly, don't take yourself too far out of your comfort zone or you'll injure yourself, burn out or develop a negative attitude and stop your program altogether. Track your workouts in writing to ensure you're progressing. Once you've achieved your cardiovascular fitness goals, then you can choose how best to maintain your fitness level.

SECTION 3: YBYL FITNESS PLAN

FUNDAMENTAL #2:
TRAIN TWO TO THREE TIMES PER WEEK FOR AT LEAST 30 MINUTES.

Choose at least two types of aerobic training that you'll do on a regular basis and alternate workouts. Also, alternate steady-state training (constant pace and intensity) with interval training (varying pace and intensity). Doing so will challenge different muscles at different angles, and allow your body to better recover between workouts. Please refer to the Appendix for sample workout programs.

If you're not ready to begin a resistance training program, then choose at least two forms of cardio-muscular training listed earlier in this section and alternate these workouts with your aerobic training.

FUNDAMENTAL #3:
TRAIN IN A WAY THAT MAXIMIZES RESULTS IN THE TIME YOU'RE INVESTING.

For most people, training aerobically for shorter periods (30 minutes) at medium to high intensity is superior to training for longer periods (40-60 minutes) at low intensity. This is particularly true for busy people. Medium to high intensity aerobic workouts take less time to achieve the same results and cause your metabolism to stay elevated long after you're done. They also release more natural human growth hormone, thus reducing your body's biological age and building and maintaining more muscle - increasing your metabolism and shaping your body. Individuals with injuries or physical limitations, those in the first four to six weeks of a fitness program, and older adults shouldn't exercise at a high-intensity. And endurance athletes will obviously need to train for longer periods.

Remember, 30 seconds of poor eating can erase 30 minutes of great cardiovascular training. Don't think that hours and hours of aerobic training will burn away all your body fat. Remember, 75 percent of your results will come from your success with your eating plan. As far as burning body fat and increasing overall fitness is concerned, pushing away non-nutritious foods is your best exercise.

SECTION 3: YBYL FITNESS PLAN

YBYL Flexibility Training

Flexibility is the amount of movement that can be achieved at a joint, such as the knee or shoulder. Inflexibility increases your risk for joint and muscle injury. As every system in your body must be challenged to make progress, so must the connective tissue and skeletal muscles so you become more flexible and properly align the body. Consistent, safe stretching and yoga practice may be conducted before, during and after workouts, or on its own. Please refer to the Appendix for YBYL Super Stretches.

THE BENEFITS OF IMPROVED FLEXIBILITY AND PHYSICAL ALIGNMENT INCLUDE:

- Increased energy and endurance
- Less risk of injury and chronic physical conditions
- Improved muscular efficiency
- Improved circulation
- Faster recovery between workouts
- Improved body shape and muscular symmetry
- Improved sports performance

A WORD ABOUT YOGA

First of all, I love yoga and, along with weight training, I know that yoga is something that I will continue to do the rest of my life. While yoga classes vary greatly, I believe a safe, effective yoga practice is beneficial to most people. However, it's important to be clear on your goals before selecting a yoga practice that's right for you.

Most American yoga classes are a variation of Hatha, where postures (asanas) range from the seemingly simple (standing erect) to the very complex (putting your feet behind your head and balancing on your hands). Challenging physical forms of Hatha yoga include: Bikram, Ashtanga or "Power" Yoga and Iyengar.

- **BIKRAM YOGA**
  is an intense workout conducted in a room heated to more than 100 degrees. This form has the major benefit of comprehensive detoxification, since you'll be sweating profusely the entire class, besides improving flexibility.

SECTION 3: YBYL FITNESS PLAN

- **ASHTANGA YOGA OR "POWER" YOGA**
  is a physically challenging series of yoga flows or vinyasas. This form follows a set series from beginning to end without stopping and is designed to create and maintain heat in the body and cleanse at the cellular level. This is one of the most physically challenging forms of yoga and is a great workout.

- **IYENGAR YOGA**
  focuses on precise attention to alignment in every pose. Basic to this practice are the standing poses, which are often held longer than they are in other styles of yoga. Props such as blocks, belts and blankets are sometimes used in Iyengar-style classes to give the body support. An Iyengar yoga class may be slow, soft and meditative, or it may be extremely challenging and physically demanding.

As with personal trainers, some yoga instructors are better than others, so find a great instructor and don't judge yoga based on only one or two experiences. One of the great things about yoga is that once you know what you're doing, you can easily practice it in your home, office, the gym or any quiet place. Remember though, your fitness program should also challenge the cardiovascular system and muscular system and, unless you're practicing a challenging form of yoga at a very high level, yoga will best serve as one part of your total fitness program.

Words cannot convey the value of Yoga. It has to be experienced.

—B.K.S. Iyengar, founder of Iyengar yoga

The Three YBYL Fundamentals of Flexibility Training:

1. Be safe and gradual, yet progressively challenge yourself until you've achieved your flexibility and physical alignment goals.
2. Stretch your entire body daily for at least 10 minutes.
3. Stretch in a way that maximizes results in the time you're investing.

SECTION 3: YBYL FITNESS PLAN

FUNDAMENTAL #1:
BE SAFE AND GRADUAL, YET PROGRESSIVELY CHALLENGE YOURSELF UNTIL YOU'VE ACHIEVED YOUR FLEXIBILITY AND PHYSICAL ALIGNMENT GOALS.

SAFE.
Develop correct form on all stretches and yoga asanas. Doing so will allow you to improve your flexibility and physical alignment, while minimizing your chance of injury. Never stretch a cold muscle; the best time to stretch is when your muscles are warm. Don't bob or bounce; a slow sustained stretch is best.

GRADUAL AND PROGRESSIVE.
Hold each stretch for 10 to 30 seconds, breathe rhythmically, and try to extend the stretch as you exhale. Slowly stretch until you feel tightness in the muscles. Slight discomfort is okay, but don't stretch to the point of pain.

FUNDAMENTAL #2:
STRETCH YOUR ENTIRE BODY DAILY FOR AT LEAST 10 MINUTES.

Depending on your flexibility, physical alignment goals and your potential for injury, you may want to stretch more or less. Stretching is also a great anti-stress activity that you can do almost anywhere, so don't limit your stretching to before, during or after workouts. Stretching or practicing yoga in the morning is a great way to start the day; stretching or practicing yoga at night is a great way to end the day.

FUNDAMENTAL #3:
STRETCH IN A WAY THAT MAXIMIZES RESULTS IN THE TIME YOU'RE INVESTING.

Whenever possible, do compound, multi-joint stretches that stretch a large percentage of your body at one time. Stretching between resistance training sets is a good idea, since your muscles are warm, and you want to catch your breath before beginning a new exercise anyway. Stretch throughout the day whenever you have some free time. Stretch frequently for short periods, especially if you spend a lot of time sitting during the day. Stretch at home while watching television or listening to music. Please refer to the Appendix for YBYL Super Stretches. If shaping your body is a priority, you should build your fitness program around resistance training, cardio-muscular training and yoga and follow the YBYL Eating Plan.

SECTION 3: YBYL FITNESS PLAN

YBYL Resistance Training

Resistance training refers to activities that significantly challenge the muscular system, e.g. weight training, and lead to improvements in muscular strength, muscular endurance and muscular shape. In the YBYL Program, muscular strength is the maximum amount of force a muscle or muscle groups can achieve during a single contraction. Muscular endurance is the number of repeated contractions a muscle or muscle group can perform against resistance without fatiguing. Muscular shaping refers to the process of increasing the amount of lean muscle mass relative to fat in any given area of the body. Muscular symmetry is the extent to which muscle groups are properly balanced in size and strength.

When trying to lose body fat, it's important to maintain or add muscle because muscle is the body's most metabolically active tissue. For every pound of muscle that you add or preserve, your body will burn an additional 50 to 75 calories per day. And, when you exercise, you burn more calories and your metabolism stays elevated longer - the more muscle you have. Thus, if you add or preserve five pounds of muscle, you can expect to burn an additional 250 to 375 calories per day, every day, without doing anything else. In addition, when you challenge your muscles, you strengthen your bones and connective tissue, release human growth hormone and turn back the clock. Without challenging your muscles on a regular basis, muscle loss, strength loss and less muscle tone is inevitable - and the primary reason our metabolism slows down as we age. The only way to know for sure that you are adding muscle is to continue to increase the amount of resistance and challenge your muscles.

When healthy people participate in resistance training, their bones become denser through increases in collagen fibers and mineral salts. However, if bones aren't subjected to stress, as with sedentary individuals, they become less dense over time as they lose mineral salts. In men, the loss of minerals may begin at age 50, but in women it may start as early as age 30. By age 70, some women may have lost 70 percent of their bone mineral mass. For this reason, resistance training is particularly important for older women because low levels of estrogen hormone lead to substantial bone mineral loss, unless the bones and muscles are challenged regularly by resistance training, cardio-muscular training or yoga. When it comes to bones and muscles, natural law is simple and unforgiving: What we don't use, we lose! What we use, we keep!

A growing body of evidence suggests that resistance training has cardiovascular benefits, including decreased bad cholesterol levels, increased efficiency within the heart and decreased blood pressure. Consistent, progressive resistance training, cardiovascular training, cardio-muscular training, flexibility training and adherence to the YBYL Eating Plan will maximize your ability to burn body fat as fuel.

PLEASE REFER TO THE APPENDIX FOR THE YBYL RESISTANCE TRAINING ROUTINE.

The Three YBYL Fundamentals of Resistance Training:

1. Be safe and gradual, yet progressively challenge yourself until you've achieved your strength and body shaping goals.
2. Train your upper and lower body at least once per week.
3. Train in a way that maximizes results in the time you're investing.

FUNDAMENTAL #1:
BE SAFE AND GRADUAL, YET PROGRESSIVELY CHALLENGE YOURSELF UNTIL YOU'VE ACHIEVED YOUR STRENGTH AND BODY SHAPING GOALS.

SAFE.

Develop correct form on all exercises. Doing so will allow you to train with high intensity while minimizing your chance of injury. If you train with high intensity and you have poor technique, your chance of injury is quite high. Working with a personal trainer who insists on perfect technique is well worth the investment, even if it's only for a few workouts so you get the hang of it. It's been my experience that 90 percent of those who lift weights in the gym have poor technique, so don't do an exercise the way someone else does it. If you don't hire a trainer, then copy someone who uses correct form.

WARM UP AND COOL DOWN.

Always warm up before working out. The purpose of the warm-up is to elevate your body temperature and blood pressure and increase the temperature of muscle and connective tissue, thereby reducing the risk of injury. Warming up also reduces the body's potential for fatigue. Cool down after working out to facilitate

SECTION 3: YBYL FITNESS PLAN

recovery. After warming up your body for at least five minutes before your workout, do one to two warm-up sets using multi-joint compound movements. Never lift weights intensely without first warming up.

GRADUAL AND PROGRESSIVE.

If you're just beginning a resistance training program, train at low to medium intensity for at least four weeks to strengthen your muscles, bones and connective tissue. After this initial period, train at medium to high intensity and take each set to muscular failure. By taking each set to muscular failure (with correct form), you will force your muscles to grow and become stronger. While reducing body fat through cardio and eating well is healthy, you need muscle to shape your body.

Resist the temptation to do the same exercises with the same weight, reps and sets. Instead, increase your weight or reps each workout on several exercises. Track your workouts in writing. Having a workout partner or trainer also helps.

A good rule of thumb is to try to make your body fairly sore after each workout. If you're really sore (for more than four or five days), you probably over-trained; if you're not sore at all, you probably under-trained. Don't resistance-train a sore body part. This is over-training, counterproductive and may lead to injury.

Once you've achieved your strength and body shaping goals, you can go for a higher level maintenance program. If you're bored with resistance training, vary your workouts, increase your intensity, and set measurable goals.

FUNDAMENTAL #2:
TRAIN YOUR UPPER AND LOWER BODY AT LEAST ONCE PER WEEK.

You need to train your entire body to achieve muscular symmetry. Based on your body's current symmetry, you may choose to spend additional time and energy on less developed areas, but you should train your upper and lower body at least once per week. Men may choose to train chest and back on one day, and legs, shoulders and arms the next. Women may want to supplement once a week lower body resistance training with a couple of days of lower body cardio-muscular training. If you want to give either your lower body or upper body more attention, then train it twice per week with at least 72 hours of recovery between workouts.

If shaping your body is a top priority, then start out with 30-minute sessions and gradually build up to 45-minute sessions. If you're not yet ready to begin resistance training, then choose at least two forms of cardio-muscular training and alternate these workouts with pure aerobic training.

FUNDAMENTAL #3:
TRAIN IN A WAY THAT MAXIMIZES RESULTS IN THE TIME YOU'RE INVESTING.

FOCUS ON MULTI-JOINT, COMPOUND MOVEMENTS.

Spend at least 75 percent of your time and energy training large muscles (legs, gluteus, back, chest and abs) with multi-joint, compound movements, and 25 percent or less training smaller muscles (arms and shoulders) with single-joint isolation movements. One reason for this is that your arms and shoulders are already doing lots of work when you train your chest and back. For example, while I may be training 20 percent of my total muscle mass when I do a set of lat pulls, I may only be training 5 percent of my muscle mass when I do a set of dumbbell curls.

TRAIN BOTH SIDES OF THE BODY AT THE SAME TIME.

When doing single-joint upper body isolation movements, train both sides of the body at the same time. Since the time you have to lift weights is limited, training one side at a time can only be justified if it is twice as effective as training both sides at the same time. For example, while I may be training 5 percent of my total muscle mass when I do a set of 2-arm dumbbell curls, I'm only training 2.5 percent of my total muscle mass when I do them individually.

VARY REPETITION SPEED.

Alternate normal resistance training (two to three seconds per rep) with slow resistance training (10 seconds per rep). Doing so will challenge your muscles at different angles in different ways, minimize overuse injuries, and allow your body to better recover between workouts. When you train at a slower speed, you'll need to decrease the amount of weight you lift. Unless you're a power lifter or striving for improved sports performance, each repetition you do should last at least two seconds. A common mistake is the tendency to lift weights too quickly and use momentum.

For normal speed upper body resistance training, increase the amount of weight once you can complete 12 or more reps. For slow speed upper body resistance training, increase the amount of weight once you can complete six or more reps. Regardless of speed, an upper body exercise set should last about 30 to 45 seconds.

For normal speed lower body resistance training, increase the amount of weight once you can complete 15 or more reps. For slow speed lower body resistance training, increase the amount of weight once you can complete 10 or more reps. A lower body exercise set should last about 45 to 60 seconds. Alternate different

SECTION 3: YBYL FITNESS PLAN

resistance training exercises every few weeks.

AVOID MOMENTUM.

Keep the appropriate muscles contracted the entire time when you do an exercise. Don't rest at the top or bottom of a movement, and don't lock your arms or legs or you'll put undue stress on your joints. Rest between sets, not between reps. Keep the speed constant throughout the movement. Don't speed up and slow down. Remember, "momentum's not your friend in the gym."

PARTIAL REPS.

Once you've completed as many full-range reps as you can with correct form, you may want to do a few partial-range reps to further exhaust the muscle.

REST TIME.

A good rule of thumb is to rest long enough to catch your breath. You'll need more rest time after a challenging set of leg presses than you will after a set of side lateral dumbbell raises.

ABDOMINAL EXERCISES.

A common mistake I see in the gym is people who are doing lots of low-intensity, high-rep ab exercises that don't effectively isolate the abs. First, I know that any high intensity resistance training exercise works your abs. Thus, the best way to train your abs is to train with high intensity on all exercises. Although your abs may recover slightly faster than some other muscles, the same training principles still apply. If your goals are to make your abs stronger and add muscle to them then, as with your lower body, your abs should fail 45 to 60 seconds after starting the exercise. The ab exercises I've included minimize hip flexion, isolate the abs and allow you to progressively increase resistance over time. I generally discourage weighted side-bends because, unless you have very low body fat, the additional muscle beneath the fat will make your waist larger, not smaller. But adding a slight twisting movement on your crunches will develop your obliques and intercostal muscles nicely.

LOWER BACK EXERCISES.

The lower back may be both the most important and the most neglected body part. Along with your abs, your lower back is your body's core. Train your abs two to three times per week and your lower back two times per week.

PLEASE REFER TO THE APPENDIX FOR THE YBYL RESISTANCE TRAINING ROUTINE.

SECTION 3: YBYL FITNESS PLAN

HOW TO FIND A GREAT PERSONAL TRAINER

It is worth your time to research and interview several personal trainers before hiring one. Here are just some of the questions you may want to ask:

- What is your weekly workout routine?
- How many times per week do you encourage clients to lift weights, and how do you split up your routines? What are your training sessions like?
- What is your eating philosophy for clients as it relates to achieving health, fitness and body shaping goals?
- What are your rates? What are your payment and cancellation policies?
- What is your athletic background? What are your education and training credentials?

You may also want to show them the YBYL Program Summary and see if they agree with the YBYL Fundamentals. If shaping your body is a priority to you, hire a trainer who is in great shape. If your trainer isn't in great shape, he will have a difficult time getting you in great shape.

HOW TO FIND A GREAT YOGA INSTRUCTOR

Since you can generally try out any yoga classes to see how you like it, finding a great yoga instructor is easier than finding a great personal trainer. At the very least, you should find a yoga instructor who takes great care of his or her body and has a regular practice. Before trying a class, you may want to:

- Decide what type of yoga you want to practice.
- Decide what days and times you can practice.
- Research all your options.
- Go to several styles of yoga classes and choose the ones you prefer.

Please Complete Section 3 Workbook Exercises Now.

Section 4: YBYL™ Workbook

SECTION 4: YBYL WORKBOOK

Overview

Your YBYL Workbook is your comprehensive action plan. By completing and reviewing this written plan, you'll greatly increase your chance of achieving your goals. Because you're replacing old, self-destructive habits that no longer serve you with new, empowering habits that will improve your life in a powerful way, a high degree of repetition and self-discipline is appropriate and necessary. After all, fuzzy goals that aren't in writing and accompanied by a plan are mere fantasies.

If you execute this program as I've designed it, I guarantee your success. Your YBYL Workbook will tell you what to do; it's up to you to do it. To the extent that you veer off of the plan and try to do it "your way," well, you're on your own. This program works if you embrace gradual change and if you also become your own success coach. If you want to be successful, then get into it! The more you get into it, the greater your success will be. Commit fully! As always, I wish you the best of luck on your quest. Enjoy the journey!

SECTION 4: YBYL WORKBOOK

Section 1: Preparing for Success

These exercises will help you develop your goals and action plan and give you total clarity regarding what you want, why you want it and what you will do to get it. Please complete these exercises with a pencil so that you can make appropriate changes.

YBYL GENERAL GOALS
- ☐ Shape my body!
- ☐ Look younger!
- ☐ Feel and perform better!
- ☐ Live longer!

1. **LIST YOUR TOP FIVE 1-MONTH GOALS.**

    1. I'll lose _____ lbs. per week and weigh _____ lbs. by ___/___/___ (date) and my waist will be _____, or I will be a size _____.

    2. I'll work out _____ days per week _____ minutes each day (on average).

    3. _____.

    4. _____.

    5. _____.

2. **LIST YOUR TOP FIVE 3-MONTH GOALS.**

    1. I'll lose _____ lbs. per week and weigh _____ lbs. by ___/___/___ (date) and my waist will be _____, or I will be a size _____.

    2. I'll work out _____ days per week _____ minutes each day (on average).

    3. _____.

    4. _____.

    5. _____.

SECTION 4: YBYL WORKBOOK   Your Body, Your Life™

3. **LIST YOUR TOP FIVE 1-YEAR GOALS.**

    1. I'll lose _____ lbs. per week and weigh _____ lbs. by ___/___/___ (date) and my waist will be _____, or I will be a size _____.

    2. I'll work out _____ days per week _____ minutes each day (on average).

    3. _____

    4. _____

    5. _____

4. **LIST THE TOP FIVE ACTIONS YOU'LL TAKE TO ACHIEVE YOUR GOALS.**

    1. _____
    2. _____
    3. _____
    4. _____
    5. _____

5. **HOW MUCH DO YOU WANT TO ACHIEVE YOUR GOALS? WHY IS THIS SO IMPORTANT TO YOU NOW? HOW SURE ARE YOU THAT YOU'LL ACHIEVE THEM? HOW COMMITTED?**

    _____
    _____
    _____
    _____
    _____

6. **LIST FIVE EXCITING REASONS WHY YOU WILL ACHIEVE YOUR GOALS.**

    1. _____
    2. _____
    3. _____
    4. _____
    5. _____

SECTION 4: YBYL WORKBOOK

7. LIST FIVE NEGATIVE CONSEQUENCES OF NOT ACHIEVING YOUR GOALS.

1. _____.
2. _____.
3. _____.
4. _____.
5. _____.

MAKE SEVERAL COPIES OF YOUR GOALS AND PUT THEM WHERE YOU CAN REVIEW THEM A FEW TIMES EACH DAY.

8. LIST FIVE OBSTACLES YOU'LL OVERCOME TO ACHIEVE YOUR GOALS.

1. Obstacle _____ Solution _____
2. Obstacle _____ Solution _____
3. Obstacle _____ Solution _____
4. Obstacle _____ Solution _____
5. Obstacle _____ Solution _____

9. LIST YOUR PAST LIMITING BELIEFS ABOUT FOOD AND EXERCISE THAT YOU'RE REPLACING WITH NEW IMPROVED BELIEFS THAT SUPPORT YOUR GOALS AND ACTION PLAN.

Old Belief : _____

New Belief : _____

Old Belief : _____

New Belief : _____

Old Belief : _____

New Belief : _____

Old Belief : _____

New Belief : _____

SECTION 4: YBYL WORKBOOK

Your Body, Your Life™

10. LIST SUPPORT PEOPLE, MENTORS, WORKOUT PARTNERS AND COACHES WHO YOU WANT TO SUPPORT YOU. (CIRCLE THEIR NAMES ONCE YOU'VE CONTACTED THEM.)

_____.
_____.
_____.

11. WHAT NEW SUCCESS RITUALS WILL YOU INTEGRATE INTO YOUR DAILY ROUTINE?

_____.
_____.
_____.

12. PLEASE CHECK THE AFFIRMATIONS THAT YOU'LL REVIEW REGULARLY.

- ☐ weigh _____ pounds and feel great.
- ☐ eat healthfully as a rule, not as an exception.
- ☐ drink a lot of water and enjoy nutritious foods every day.
- ☐ eat three small/moderate meals per day and two snacks.
- ☐ never feel either famished or extremely full.
- ☐ plan ahead and take nutritious foods with me.
- ☐ I'm healthy, lean and fit.
- ☐ I'm willing and able to pay a price to achieve my goals.
- ☐ love, admire and respect my body.
- ☐ Working out and exercising is a vital part of my life.
- ☐ overcome all challenges that come my way.
- ☐ visualize my success and how it makes me feel.
- ☐ focus on what I want, not on what I don't want.
- ☐ enjoy taking the steps to achieve my goals.
- ☐ take responsibility for my actions.
- ☐ _____.
- ☐ _____.
- ☐ _____.

SECTION 4: YBYL WORKBOOK

13. PLEASE CHECK THE SUCCESS DISCIPLINES THAT YOU'LL EMPLOY.

- ☐ Pray and ask God for His help and support.
- ☐ Review and update my goals and action plan at least once a week.
- ☐ Think and talk positively and confidently.
- ☐ Transform relevant values and beliefs so that they support achieving my goals.
- ☐ Implement Success Rituals.
- ☐ Organize, plan and employ self-discipline.
- ☐ Make steady, gradual improvements in my eating and exercise habits.
- ☐ View food primarily as fuel.
- ☐ Visualize my success. When? _____
  How often? _____
- ☐ Read positive affirmations. When? _____
  How often? _____
- ☐ Post my goals and put up inspirational pictures.
  Where? _____
- ☐ Cultivate support people, workout partners, mentors, trainers and coaches.
- ☐ Write in a success journal. When? _____
  How often? _____
- ☐ Cultivate anti-stress activities. What? _____
- ☐ Personal Strategic Planning. When? _____
- ☐ Use YBYL Weekly Training Logs and the YBYL Action Item Form.
- ☐ Complete the YBYL 28-Day Jumpstart Program.

Please Read Section 2 of YBYL

SECTION 4: YBYL WORKBOOK

Your Body, Your Life™

Section 2: YBYL Eating Plan

TO LOSE ONE POUND OF BODY FAT PER WEEK, YOU MUST BURN 500 CALORIES PER DAY MORE THAN YOU CONSUME.

1. ☐ READ SECTION 2 OF YBYL. (CHECK WHEN COMPLETED.)

2. **DETERMINING YOUR OPTIMUM DAILY CALORIC INTAKE.**

   Although the formula below isn't appropriate for everyone because of variations in lean muscle, daily caloric expenditure, and other factors, it's a good starting point for most people.

   ☐ If you want to lose bodyweight, multiply your weight by 10.
   Your weight _____ x 10 = _____
   (optimum daily calories for weight loss)

   ☐ If you want to maintain your weight, multiply your weight by 15.
   Your weight _____ x 15 = _____
   (optimum daily maintenance calories)

   ☐ To determine the approximate amount of weight you would lose weekly if you followed this plan perfectly, subtract the top number from the bottom number. This is your net daily calories burned. Multiply this number by seven to determine net weekly calories burned. Divide by 3,500 to determine the number of pounds you would lose per week.

   Example: 200 pound man who wants to lose weight

2,000 Calories	=	Optimum daily calories for weight loss
3,000 Calories	=	Optimum daily maintenance calories
1,000 Calories	=	Net daily calories burned
7,000 Calories	=	Net weekly calories burned
2 pounds	=	number of pounds he would lose weekly

   Note: Rapid initial weight loss may occur due to decreased carbohydrate and sodium consumption and increased water and fiber consumption.

Your Body, Your Life™ SECTION 4: YBYL WORKBOOK

3. **DETERMINING YOUR OPTIMUM MEAL AND SNACK CALORIES, ASSUMING THREE MEALS AND TWO SNACKS PER DAY.**

   ☐ Optimum daily calories _____ x .75 = _____ (Total daily meal calories)

   ☐ Total daily meal calories _____ ÷ 3 = _____ (Optimum meal calories)

   ☐ Optimum daily calories _____ x .25 = _____ (Total daily snack calories)

   ☐ Total daily meal calories _____ ÷ 2 = _____ (Optimum snack calories)

4. **DETERMINING OPTIMUM PROTEIN-CARB-FAT AMOUNTS.**

   From the three options below, please choose the plan that you believe is right for you.

   ☐ **40% PROTEIN, 30% CARBOHYDRATES AND 30% FAT**
   works well if you are ... trying to lose body fat, fairly sensitive to carbs, used to watching your carb intake, fairly active and work out with medium intensity two to five days per week, want to reduce water retention by reducing carb consumption.

   ☐ **40% PROTEIN, 40% CARBOHYDRATES AND 20% FAT**
   works well if you are ... trying to lose body fat, not very sensitive to carbs (they don't create a substantial rise in blood sugar), used to watching fat intake, active and work out intensely four to six days per week.

   ☐ **30% PROTEIN, 50% CARBOHYDRATES AND 20% FAT**
   works well if you are ... trying to maintain your current weight and body fat level, not sensitive to carbs, a vegetarian, active and work out with intensity four to six days per week or are a competitive athlete.

   * You may also opt for the ratio that Barry Sears recommends in *The Zone*. Just make sure you don't consume too many calories.

5. **REFER TO THE APPENDIX TO DETERMINE YOUR SPECIFIC PROTEIN-CARB-FAT AMOUNTS.**

   ☐ _____ = Total optimum daily calories

   ☐ _____ = Optimum per-meal calories

   ☐ _____ = Optimum per-snack calories

   ☐ _____ = Optimum daily protein (in grams)

   ☐ _____ = Optimum daily carbs (in grams)

   ☐ _____ = Optimum daily fat (in grams)

www.ybyl.com

SECTION 4: YBYL WORKBOOK

Your Body, Your Life™

OPTIMUM PER-MEAL PROTEIN-CARB-FAT AMOUNTS

☐ _____ grams of protein

☐ _____ grams of carbs

☐ _____ grams of fat

OPTIMUM PER-SNACK PROTEIN-CARB-FAT AMOUNTS

☐ _____ grams of protein

☐ _____ grams of carbs

☐ _____ grams of fat

6. **DETERMINING YOUR OPTIMUM AMOUNTS OF WATER, FIBER AND SODIUM.**

    ☐ _____ ounces = Optimum water per day (.75 x weight ... this is a minimum)

    ☐ _____ grams = Optimum fiber per day (weight / 6 ... this is a minimum.)

    ☐ _____ mg = Optimum sodium per day (weight x 10)

7. ☐ **REVIEW YBYL FOOD PYRAMID IN THE APPENDIX AND CHECK OFF FOODS THAT YOU'LL INCLUDE IN YOUR EATING PLAN. DO THE SAME FOR OTHER FAMILY MEMBERS.** (CHECK WHEN COMPLETED.)

8. ☐ **REVIEW YBYL DETOX PLAN IN THE APPENDIX.** (CHECK WHEN COMPLETED.)

9. ☐ **REVIEW YBYL SUPER FOODS LIST IN THE APPENDIX.** (CHECK WHEN COMPLETED.)

10. ☐ **REVIEW YBYL GROCERY LIST IN THE APPENDIX.** (CHECK WHEN COMPLETED.)

11. ☐ **USING YOUR YBYL GROCERY LIST, GO GROCERY SHOPPING AFTER A NUTRITIOUS MEAL.** (CHECK WHEN COMPLETED.)

12. ☐ **REMOVE NON-NUTRITIOUS FOODS FROM HOME AND OFFICE; MAKE NUTRITIOUS FOODS EASILY AVAILABLE.** (CHECK WHEN COMPLETED.)

SECTION 4: YBYL WORKBOOK

13. **LIST 5 FOODS THAT WILL BE CHALLENGING TO REDUCE OR ELIMINATE FROM YOUR DIET, AND A BETTER OPTION FOR EACH ONE.**

   1. _____

      Better option: _____

   2. _____

      Better option: _____

   3. _____

      Better option: _____

   4. _____

      Better option: _____

   5. _____

      Better option: _____

14. **ALCOHOL:**
   - List the maximum number of drinks, glasses of wine or beer that you'll consume per week: _____.
   - Total alcohol-related calories: _____.

15. **PLEASE LIST THE NUTRITIONAL SUPPLEMENTS THAT YOU'LL TAKE DAILY AND WHEN YOU'LL TAKE THEM.**

   _____.
   _____.
   _____.
   _____.

16. **PLEASE USE THE YBYL ACTION ITEM FORM AT THE END OF THE WORKBOOK TO HELP YOU EXECUTE YOUR PLAN AND REVIEW THIS WORKBOOK ON A REGULAR BASIS.**

Please Read Section 3 of YBYL.

SECTION 4: YBYL WORKBOOK   *Your Body, Your Life*™

Section 3: YBYL Fitness Plan

1. ☐ **READ SECTION 3 OF YBYL.** (CHECK WHEN COMPLETED.)

2. **LIST FIVE OBSTACLES YOU'LL OVERCOME TO STAY ON YOUR FITNESS PROGRAM.**

    1. _____.
    2. _____.
    3. _____.
    4. _____.
    5. _____.

3. **REFERRING TO THE SAMPLE WORKOUT PLANS IN THE APPENDIX, DETERMINE YOUR INITIAL WORKOUT PLAN AND UPDATE REGULARLY.**

    INITIAL WORKOUT PLAN:

    Please include what, when and how much.

    MON _____
    TUE _____
    WED _____
    THU _____
    FRI _____
    SAT _____
    SUN _____

4. ☐ **SCHEDULE THESE DAYS AND TIMES IN YOUR PLANNER.** (CHECK WHEN COMPLETED.)

www.ybyl.com

SECTION 4: YBYL WORKBOOK

5. **WHAT OTHER ACTIONS WILL YOU TAKE TO ENSURE YOUR SUCCESS?**

    1. _____
    2. _____
    3. _____
    4. _____
    5. _____

6. **IF YOUR TIME IS LIMITED, WHAT ACTIVITIES WILL YOU ELIMINATE TO CREATE FIVE HOURS TO COMMIT TO YOUR FITNESS PROGRAM? ARE YOU WILLING TO GET UP EARLIER IN THE MORNING?**

    - _____
    - _____
    - _____
    - _____
    - _____

7. **WILL YOU HIRE A PERSONAL FITNESS TRAINER EITHER FOR SHORT-TERM HELP OR LONG-TERM SUPPORT? IF SO, WHAT IS YOUR PLAN FOR FINDING A GREAT TRAINER?**

    - _____
    - _____
    - _____
    - _____
    - _____

SECTION 4: YBYL WORKBOOK

Your Body, Your Life™

YBYL ACTION ITEMS AND CRITICAL SUCCESS FACTORS
(PLEASE LIST AND CHECK WHEN COMPLETED.)

- [ ] _____.
- [ ] _____.
- [ ] _____.
- [ ] _____.
- [ ] _____.
- [ ] _____.
- [ ] _____.
- [ ] _____.
- [ ] _____.
- [ ] _____.
- [ ] _____.
- [ ] _____.
- [ ] _____.
- [ ] _____.
- [ ] _____.
- [ ] _____.
- [ ] _____.
- [ ] _____.
- [ ] _____.
- [ ] _____.
- [ ] _____.
- [ ] _____.
- [ ] _____.
- [ ] _____.
- [ ] _____.
- [ ] _____.

Section 5:
YBYL™ Appendix

SECTION 5: APPENDIX

Your Body. Your Life.™

YBYL - Weekly Training Log

Name: _Michelle Sample_ Date: _10_ / _14_ / _02_ Week: _1_ of _4_

YOUR GOALS:

1. Live to be _100_ years old!
2. Weigh _130_ lbs. and be a size _6_ by _January 4, 2003_.
3. Feel and Perform at my max!
4. _Lose .75 lb per week for 12 weeks. (9 lbs)_
5. _Shape and tone my entire body!_

YOUR DAILY EATING GOALS:

Daily: _1,500_ cal, **3 meals, 2 snacks,** _40_ % prot., _30_ % carb, _30_ % fat

Meal Goal: _375_ cal, _38_ g protein, _28_ g carb, _13_ g fat

Snack Goal: _188_ cal, _19_ g protein, _14_ g carb, _7_ g fat

Water Goal: _128 oz_ Fiber Goal: _25 g_ Sodium Goal: _< 1400 mg_

YOUR WEEKLY EXERCISE GOALS:

Average Exercise Goal: _45_ minutes per day, _6_ days per week

Exercise Goal Specifics: _Weights - 2x, Cardio - 2x, Yoga class - 2x_

CHECK THE SUCCESS DISCIPLINES YOU PRACTICED:

- ☐ Prayed and asked God for His help and support
- ☐ Thought and talked positively
- ☐ Transformed disempowering values and beliefs to empowering ones
- ☐ Implemented success rituals and routines
- ☐ Organized, planned and employed self-discipline
- ☐ Embraced positive accountability
- ☐ Made steady, gradual improvements in my eating and exercise habits
- ☐ Viewed food as fuel
- ☐ Read and wrote out positive affirmations
- ☐ Visualized my success
- ☐ Displayed inspirational pictures
- ☐ Cultivated support people, workout partners, mentors, coaches and trainers
- ☐ Wrote in a success journal
- ☐ Cultivated stress-reducing activities
- ☐ Did personal strategic planning

www.ybyl.com

SECTION 5: APPENDIX

ACTUAL EXERCISE AND FOOD CONSUMPTION:

DAY	DATE	EXERCISE			BODY WEIGHT
Mon	10/14	45 min / weights, lower body			
WATER (oz)	FIBER (g)	EST. CALORIES	PROTIEN (g)	CARBS (g)	FAT (g)
128 oz	30 g	1800 cal	150 g	160 g	60 g
DAY	DATE	EXERCISE			BODY WEIGHT
Tue	10/15	75 min. / yoga, light			
WATER (oz)	FIBER (g)	EST. CALORIES	PROTIEN (g)	CARBS (g)	FAT (g)
96 oz	25 g	1200 cal	150 g	60 g	40 g
DAY	DATE	EXERCISE			BODY WEIGHT
Wed	10/16	30 min. / walk at incline			
WATER (oz)	FIBER (g)	EST. CALORIES	PROTIEN (g)	CARBS (g)	FAT (g)
144 oz	32 g	1500 cal	150 g	113 g	50 g
DAY	DATE	EXERCISE			BODY WEIGHT
Thu	10/17	30 min. / weights, upper body			
WATER (oz)	FIBER (g)	EST. CALORIES	PROTIEN (g)	CARBS (g)	FAT (g)
84 oz	16 g	1800 cal	180 g	130 g	60 g
DAY	DATE	EXERCISE			BODY WEIGHT
Fri	10/18	30 min. / stair machine			
WATER (oz)	FIBER (g)	EST. CALORIES	PROTIEN (g)	CARBS (g)	FAT (g)
144 oz	25 g	1200 cal	120 g	90 g	40 g
DAY	DATE	EXERCISE			BODY WEIGHT
Sat	10/19	75 min. / yoga, light			
WATER (oz)	FIBER (g)	EST. CALORIES	PROTIEN (g)	CARBS (g)	FAT (g)
128 oz	23 g	1500 cal	150 g	113 g	50 g
DAY	DATE	EXERCISE			BODY WEIGHT
Sun	10/20	rest and recovery			
WATER (oz)	FIBER (g)	EST. CALORIES	PROTIEN (g)	CARBS (g)	FAT (g)
128 oz	30 g	1800 cal	180 g	130 g	60 g

COMMENTS / JOURNAL / ACTION ITEMS:

This was the first week of the Jumpstart Program and I'm off to a great start! Having a protein shake and a protein bar a day is helping keep the protein intake up and my blood sugar level steady. I feel great!

SECTION 5: APPENDIX

Your Body, Your Life™

YBYL - Weekly Training Log: 28-day Jumpstart

Name: _____ Date: ___/___/___ Week: _1_ of _4_

YOUR GOALS:

1. Live to be _____ years old!
2. Weigh _____ lbs. and be a size _____ by _____.
3. Feel and Perform at my max!
4. _____
5. _____

YOUR DAILY EATING GOALS:

Daily: _____ cal, **3 meals**, **2 snacks**, ____% prot., ____% carb, ____% fat

Meal Goal: _____ cal, _____ g protein, _____ g carb, _____ g fat

Snack Goal: _____ cal, _____ g protein, _____ g carb, _____ g fat

Water Goal: _____ Fiber Goal: _____ Sodium Goal: _____

YOUR WEEKLY EXERCISE GOALS:

Average Exercise Goal: _____ minutes per day, _____ days per week

Exercise Goal Specifics: _____

CHECK THE SUCCESS DISCIPLINES YOU PRACTICED:

- ☐ Prayed and asked God for His help and support
- ☐ Thought and talked positively
- ☐ Transformed disempowering values and beliefs to empowering ones
- ☐ Implemented success rituals and routines
- ☐ Organized, planned and employed self-discipline
- ☐ Embraced positive accountability
- ☐ Made steady, gradual improvements in my eating and exercise habits
- ☐ Viewed food as fuel
- ☐ Read and wrote out positive affirmations
- ☐ Visualized my success
- ☐ Displayed inspirational pictures
- ☐ Cultivated support people, workout partners, mentors, coaches and trainers
- ☐ Wrote in a success journal
- ☐ Cultivated stress-reducing activities
- ☐ Did personal strategic planning

www.ybyl.com

SECTION 5: APPENDIX

ACTUAL EXERCISE AND FOOD CONSUMPTION:

DAY	DATE	EXERCISE	BODY WEIGHT
WATER (oz)	FIBER (g)	EST. CALORIES	PROTIEN (g)	CARBS (g)	FAT (g)

DAY	DATE	EXERCISE	BODY WEIGHT
WATER (oz)	FIBER (g)	EST. CALORIES	PROTIEN (g)	CARBS (g)	FAT (g)

DAY	DATE	EXERCISE	BODY WEIGHT
WATER (oz)	FIBER (g)	EST. CALORIES	PROTIEN (g)	CARBS (g)	FAT (g)

DAY	DATE	EXERCISE	BODY WEIGHT
WATER (oz)	FIBER (g)	EST. CALORIES	PROTIEN (g)	CARBS (g)	FAT (g)

DAY	DATE	EXERCISE	BODY WEIGHT
WATER (oz)	FIBER (g)	EST. CALORIES	PROTIEN (g)	CARBS (g)	FAT (g)

DAY	DATE	EXERCISE	BODY WEIGHT
WATER (oz)	FIBER (g)	EST. CALORIES	PROTIEN (g)	CARBS (g)	FAT (g)

DAY	DATE	EXERCISE	BODY WEIGHT
WATER (oz)	FIBER (g)	EST. CALORIES	PROTIEN (g)	CARBS (g)	FAT (g)

COMMENTS / JOURNAL / ACTION ITEMS:

SECTION 5: APPENDIX

Your Body, Your Life™

YBYL - Weekly Training Log: 28-day Jumpstart

Name: _____ Date: ___/___/___ Week: _2_ of _4_

YOUR GOALS:

1. Live to be _____ years old!
2. Weigh _____ lbs. and be a size _____ by _____.
3. Feel and Perform at my max!
4. _____
5. _____

YOUR DAILY EATING GOALS:

Daily: _____ cal, **3 meals**, **2 snacks**, ____% prot., ____% carb., ____% fat

Meal Goal: _____ cal, _____ g protein, _____ g carb, _____ g fat

Snack Goal: _____ cal, _____ g protein, _____ g carb, _____ g fat

Water Goal: _____ Fiber Goal: _____ Sodium Goal: _____

YOUR WEEKLY EXERCISE GOALS:

Average Exercise Goal: _____ minutes per day, _____ days per week

Exercise Goal Specifics: _____

CHECK THE SUCCESS DISCIPLINES YOU PRACTICED:

- ☐ Prayed and asked God for His help and support
- ☐ Thought and talked positively
- ☐ Transformed disempowering values and beliefs to empowering ones
- ☐ Implemented success rituals and routines
- ☐ Organized, planned and employed self-discipline
- ☐ Embraced positive accountability
- ☐ Made steady, gradual improvements in my eating and exercise habits
- ☐ Viewed food as fuel
- ☐ Read and wrote out positive affirmations
- ☐ Visualized my success
- ☐ Displayed inspirational pictures
- ☐ Cultivated support people, workout partners, mentors, coaches and trainers
- ☐ Wrote in a success journal
- ☐ Cultivated stress-reducing activities
- ☐ Did personal strategic planning

ACTUAL EXERCISE AND FOOD CONSUMPTION:

DAY	DATE	EXERCISE	BODY WEIGHT
WATER (oz)	FIBER (g)	EST. CALORIES	PROTIEN (g)	CARBS (g)	FAT (g)

DAY	DATE	EXERCISE	BODY WEIGHT
WATER (oz)	FIBER (g)	EST. CALORIES	PROTIEN (g)	CARBS (g)	FAT (g)

DAY	DATE	EXERCISE	BODY WEIGHT
WATER (oz)	FIBER (g)	EST. CALORIES	PROTIEN (g)	CARBS (g)	FAT (g)

DAY	DATE	EXERCISE	BODY WEIGHT
WATER (oz)	FIBER (g)	EST. CALORIES	PROTIEN (g)	CARBS (g)	FAT (g)

DAY	DATE	EXERCISE	BODY WEIGHT
WATER (oz)	FIBER (g)	EST. CALORIES	PROTIEN (g)	CARBS (g)	FAT (g)

DAY	DATE	EXERCISE	BODY WEIGHT
WATER (oz)	FIBER (g)	EST. CALORIES	PROTIEN (g)	CARBS (g)	FAT (g)

DAY	DATE	EXERCISE	BODY WEIGHT
WATER (oz)	FIBER (g)	EST. CALORIES	PROTIEN (g)	CARBS (g)	FAT (g)

COMMENTS / JOURNAL / ACTION ITEMS:

SECTION 5: APPENDIX

Your Body, Your Life™

YBYL – Weekly Training Log: 28-day Jumpstart

Name: _____ Date: ___/___/___ Week: _3_ of _4_

YOUR GOALS:

1. Live to be _____ years old!
2. Weigh _____ lbs. and be a size _____ by _____.
3. Feel and Perform at my max!
4. _____
5. _____

YOUR DAILY EATING GOALS:

Daily: _____ cal, **3 meals, 2 snacks**, ____% prot., ____% carb, ____% fat

Meal Goal: _____ cal, _____ g protein, _____ g carb, _____ g fat

Snack Goal: _____ cal, _____ g protein, _____ g carb, _____ g fat

Water Goal: _____ Fiber Goal: _____ Sodium Goal: _____

YOUR WEEKLY EXERCISE GOALS:

Average Exercise Goal: _____ minutes per day, _____ days per week

Exercise Goal Specifics: _____

CHECK THE SUCCESS DISCIPLINES YOU PRACTICED:

- ☐ Prayed and asked God for His help and support
- ☐ Thought and talked positively
- ☐ Transformed disempowering values and beliefs to empowering ones
- ☐ Implemented success rituals and routines
- ☐ Organized, planned and employed self-discipline
- ☐ Embraced positive accountability
- ☐ Made steady, gradual improvements in my eating and exercise habits
- ☐ Viewed food as fuel
- ☐ Read and wrote out positive affirmations
- ☐ Visualized my success
- ☐ Displayed inspirational pictures
- ☐ Cultivated support people, workout partners, mentors, coaches and trainers
- ☐ Wrote in a success journal
- ☐ Cultivated stress-reducing activities
- ☐ Did personal strategic planning

SECTION 5: APPENDIX

ACTUAL EXERCISE AND FOOD CONSUMPTION:

DAY	DATE	EXERCISE				BODY WEIGHT
WATER (oz)	FIBER (g)	EST. CALORIES	PROTIEN (g)	CARBS (g)		FAT (g)

DAY	DATE	EXERCISE				BODY WEIGHT
WATER (oz)	FIBER (g)	EST. CALORIES	PROTIEN (g)	CARBS (g)		FAT (g)

DAY	DATE	EXERCISE				BODY WEIGHT
WATER (oz)	FIBER (g)	EST. CALORIES	PROTIEN (g)	CARBS (g)		FAT (g)

DAY	DATE	EXERCISE				BODY WEIGHT
WATER (oz)	FIBER (g)	EST. CALORIES	PROTIEN (g)	CARBS (g)		FAT (g)

DAY	DATE	EXERCISE				BODY WEIGHT
WATER (oz)	FIBER (g)	EST. CALORIES	PROTIEN (g)	CARBS (g)		FAT (g)

DAY	DATE	EXERCISE				BODY WEIGHT
WATER (oz)	FIBER (g)	EST. CALORIES	PROTIEN (g)	CARBS (g)		FAT (g)

DAY	DATE	EXERCISE				BODY WEIGHT
WATER (oz)	FIBER (g)	EST. CALORIES	PROTIEN (g)	CARBS (g)		FAT (g)

COMMENTS / JOURNAL / ACTION ITEMS:

_____

_____

_____

_____

_____

SECTION 5: APPENDIX

Your Body, Your Life™

YBYL – Weekly Training Log: 28-day Jumpstart

Name: _____ Date: ____/____/____ Week: __4__ of __4__

YOUR GOALS:

1. Live to be _____ years old!
2. Weigh _____ lbs. and be a size _____ by _____.
3. Feel and Perform at my max!
4. _____
5. _____

YOUR DAILY EATING GOALS:

Daily: _____ cal, **3 meals, 2 snacks**, _____% prot., _____% carb, _____% fat

Meal Goal: _____ cal, _____ g protein, _____ g carb, _____ g fat

Snack Goal: _____ cal, _____ g protein, _____ g carb, _____ g fat

Water Goal: _____ Fiber Goal: _____ Sodium Goal: _____

YOUR WEEKLY EXERCISE GOALS:

Average Exercise Goal: _____ minutes per day, _____ days per week

Exercise Goal Specifics: _____

CHECK THE SUCCESS DISCIPLINES YOU PRACTICED:

- ☐ Prayed and asked God for His help and support
- ☐ Thought and talked positively
- ☐ Transformed disempowering values and beliefs to empowering ones
- ☐ Implemented success rituals and routines
- ☐ Organized, planned and employed self-discipline
- ☐ Embraced positive accountability
- ☐ Made steady, gradual improvements in my eating and exercise habits
- ☐ Viewed food as fuel
- ☐ Read and wrote out positive affirmations
- ☐ Visualized my success
- ☐ Displayed inspirational pictures
- ☐ Cultivated support people, workout partners, mentors, coaches and trainers
- ☐ Wrote in a success journal
- ☐ Cultivated stress-reducing activities
- ☐ Did personal strategic planning

SECTION 5: APPENDIX

ACTUAL EXERCISE AND FOOD CONSUMPTION:

DAY	DATE	EXERCISE				BODY WEIGHT
WATER (oz)	FIBER (g)	EST. CALORIES	PROTIEN (g)	CARBS (g)		FAT (g)
DAY	DATE	EXERCISE				BODY WEIGHT
WATER (oz)	FIBER (g)	EST. CALORIES	PROTIEN (g)	CARBS (g)		FAT (g)
DAY	DATE	EXERCISE				BODY WEIGHT
WATER (oz)	FIBER (g)	EST. CALORIES	PROTIEN (g)	CARBS (g)		FAT (g)
DAY	DATE	EXERCISE				BODY WEIGHT
WATER (oz)	FIBER (g)	EST. CALORIES	PROTIEN (g)	CARBS (g)		FAT (g)
DAY	DATE	EXERCISE				BODY WEIGHT
WATER (oz)	FIBER (g)	EST. CALORIES	PROTIEN (g)	CARBS (g)		FAT (g)
DAY	DATE	EXERCISE				BODY WEIGHT
WATER (oz)	FIBER (g)	EST. CALORIES	PROTIEN (g)	CARBS (g)		FAT (g)
DAY	DATE	EXERCISE				BODY WEIGHT
WATER (oz)	FIBER (g)	EST. CALORIES	PROTIEN (g)	CARBS (g)		FAT (g)

COMMENTS / JOURNAL / ACTION ITEMS:

_____

_____

_____

_____

_____

www.ybyl.com

SECTION 5: APPENDIX

Your Body, Your Life™

YBYL - Program Summary

YBYL SEVEN STEP GOAL SETTING

1. Set clear, exciting, measurable goals, put them in writing, and decide when you'll achieve them.
2. Understand why you want to achieve your goals.
3. Commit fully to your goals, and believe that you'll achieve them.
4. Develop a comprehensive written action plan.
5. Take action every day towards your goals.
6. Measure your progress and continually improve your action plan.
7. Continually re-commit to your goals and action plan.

16 YBYL SUCCESS DISCIPLINES

1. Think and talk positively.
2. Transform ineffective values and beliefs to empowering ones.
3. Implement success rituals and routines.
4. Accept that eating nutritiously and exercising regularly requires organization, planning and self-discipline.
5. Embrace positive accountability.
6. Make steady, gradual improvements in your eating and exercise habits, not radical ones.
7. View food primarily as fuel, not as pleasure.
8. Read – and then write down – positive affirmations.
9. Visualize your success.
10. Display inspirational pictures.
11. Cultivate "support staff": workout partners, mentors, coaches, trainers, family and friends.
12. Pray and ask God for His help.
13. Start a "success journal."
14. Cultivate stress-reducing activities.
15. Complete the YBYL 28-Day Jumpstart.
16. Do personal strategic planning on Saturday or Sunday.

YBYL SEVEN CHALLENGES TO YOUR FITNESS SUCCESS

1. Most people haven't made their fitness program a priority and truly committed to it.
2. Most people associate pain and discomfort with the idea of working out regularly.
3. Most people haven't set compelling, measurable fitness goals and written them down.
4. Most people don't have an effective plan that will help them achieve their goals.
5. Most people try to go it alone and do it all themselves.
6. Most people don't eat nutritiously enough to have the energy to work out regularly.
7. Our culture is conspiring against you.

www.ybyl.com

SECTION 5: APPENDIX

THE FIVE YBYL EATING FUNDAMENTALS
1. Eat the right amount of daily calories that are optimum for achieving your goals.
2. Eat three small or moderate meals and two or three snacks daily.
3. Eat the right amount of protein, carbohydrates and fat that are optimum for achieving your goals.
4. Consume optimum amounts of water, fiber and sodium.
5. Get most of your calories from YBYL Super Foods.

THE YBYL TOP FIVE SUPPLEMENTS:
1. Water.
2. High-quality multiple vitamin-mineral supplements.
3. Pure wheat bran and soluble fiber supplements.
4. Additional antioxidants (Vitamins A, C, E, selenium, grapeseed extract, green tea).
5. Additional minerals for most adults (calcium, magnesium, zinc, etc.).

THE FIVE YBYL FUNDAMENTALS OF FITNESS TRAINING
1. Implement a fitness program that's safe, gradual, progressive, specific and scheduled.
2. Exercise four to five times per week.
3. Follow a customized fitness program that's based on achieving your specific health, fitness, body shaping and sport-specific goals.
4. Implement a well-rounded fitness program that challenges the cardiovascular system, builds muscular strength, endurance and symmetry, and increases flexibility and physical alignment.
5. Implement an efficient fitness program that maximizes results in the time you're investing.

THE THREE YBYL FUNDAMENTALS OF CARDIOVASCULAR TRAINING
1. Be safe and gradual, yet progressively challenge yourself until you've achieved your desired level of aerobic fitness.
2. Train two to three times per week for at least 30 minutes.
3. Train in a way that maximizes results in the time you're investing.

THE THREE YBYL FUNDAMENTALS OF FLEXIBILITY TRAINING
1. Be safe and gradual, yet progressively challenge yourself until you've achieved your flexibility and physical alignment goals.
2. Stretch your entire body daily for at least 10 minutes.
3. Stretch in a way that maximizes results in the time you're investing.

THE THREE YBYL FUNDAMENTALS OF RESISTANCE TRAINING
1. Be safe and gradual, yet progressively challenge yourself until you've achieved your strength and body shaping goals.
2. Train your upper and lower body at least once per week.
3. Train in a way that maximizes results in the time you're investing.

www.ybyl.com

SECTION 5: APPENDIX *Your Body, Your Life*™

YBYL – Weekly Training Log

Name: _____ Date: ___/___/___ Week: ___ of ___

YOUR GOALS:

1. Live to be _____ years old!
2. Weigh _____ lbs. and be a size _____ by _____.
3. Feel and Perform at my max!
4. _____
5. _____

YOUR DAILY EATING GOALS:

Daily: _____ cal, **3 meals, 2 snacks,** ____% prot., ____% carb., ____% fat

Meal Goal: _____ cal, _____ g protein, _____ g carb, _____ g fat

Snack Goal: _____ cal, _____ g protein, _____ g carb, _____ g fat

Water Goal: _____ Fiber Goal: _____ Sodium Goal: _____

YOUR WEEKLY EXERCISE GOALS:

Average Exercise Goal: _____ minutes per day, _____ days per week

Exercise Goal Specifics: _____

CHECK THE SUCCESS DISCIPLINES YOU PRACTICED:

- ☐ Prayed and asked God for His help and support
- ☐ Thought and talked positively
- ☐ Transformed disempowering values and beliefs to empowering ones
- ☐ Implemented success rituals and routines
- ☐ Organized, planned and employed self-discipline
- ☐ Embraced positive accountability
- ☐ Made steady, gradual improvements in my eating and exercise habits
- ☐ Viewed food as fuel
- ☐ Read and wrote out positive affirmations
- ☐ Visualized my success
- ☐ Displayed inspirational pictures
- ☐ Cultivated support people, workout partners, mentors, coaches and trainers
- ☐ Wrote in a success journal
- ☐ Cultivated stress-reducing activities
- ☐ Did personal strategic planning

www.ybyl.com

SECTION 5: APPENDIX

ACTUAL EXERCISE AND FOOD CONSUMPTION:

DAY	DATE	EXERCISE				BODY WEIGHT
WATER (oz)	FIBER (g)	EST. CALORIES	PROTIEN (g)	CARBS (g)	FAT (g)	
DAY	DATE	EXERCISE				BODY WEIGHT
WATER (oz)	FIBER (g)	EST. CALORIES	PROTIEN (g)	CARBS (g)	FAT (g)	
DAY	DATE	EXERCISE				BODY WEIGHT
WATER (oz)	FIBER (g)	EST. CALORIES	PROTIEN (g)	CARBS (g)	FAT (g)	
DAY	DATE	EXERCISE				BODY WEIGHT
WATER (oz)	FIBER (g)	EST. CALORIES	PROTIEN (g)	CARBS (g)	FAT (g)	
DAY	DATE	EXERCISE				BODY WEIGHT
WATER (oz)	FIBER (g)	EST. CALORIES	PROTIEN (g)	CARBS (g)	FAT (g)	
DAY	DATE	EXERCISE				BODY WEIGHT
WATER (oz)	FIBER (g)	EST. CALORIES	PROTIEN (g)	CARBS (g)	FAT (g)	
DAY	DATE	EXERCISE				BODY WEIGHT
WATER (oz)	FIBER (g)	EST. CALORIES	PROTIEN (g)	CARBS (g)	FAT (g)	

COMMENTS / JOURNAL / ACTION ITEMS:

_____

_____

_____

_____

_____

www.ybyl.com

SECTION 5: APPENDIX   Your Body, Your Life™

YBYL - Weekly Training Log

Name: _____ Date: ___/___/___ Week: ___ of ___

YOUR GOALS:

1. Live to be _____ years old!
2. Weigh _____ lbs. and be a size _____ by _____.
3. Feel and Perform at my max!
4. _____
5. _____

YOUR DAILY EATING GOALS:

Daily: _____ cal, **3 meals**, **2 snacks**, ____% prot., ____% carb, ____% fat

Meal Goal: _____ cal, _____ g protein, _____ g carb, _____ g fat

Snack Goal: _____ cal, _____ g protein, _____ g carb, _____ g fat

Water Goal: _____ Fiber Goal: _____ Sodium Goal: _____

YOUR WEEKLY EXERCISE GOALS:

Average Exercise Goal: _____ minutes per day, _____ days per week

Exercise Goal Specifics: _____

CHECK THE SUCCESS DISCIPLINES YOU PRACTICED:

- ☐ Prayed and asked God for His help and support
- ☐ Thought and talked positively
- ☐ Transformed disempowering values and beliefs to empowering ones
- ☐ Implemented success rituals and routines
- ☐ Organized, planned and employed self-discipline
- ☐ Embraced positive accountability
- ☐ Made steady, gradual improvements in my eating and exercise habits
- ☐ Viewed food as fuel
- ☐ Read and wrote out positive affirmations
- ☐ Visualized my success
- ☐ Displayed inspirational pictures
- ☐ Cultivated support people, workout partners, mentors, coaches and trainers
- ☐ Wrote in a success journal
- ☐ Cultivated stress-reducing activities
- ☐ Did personal strategic planning

www.ybyl.com

SECTION 5: APPENDIX

ACTUAL EXERCISE AND FOOD CONSUMPTION:

DAY	DATE	EXERCISE				BODY WEIGHT
WATER (oz)	FIBER (g)	EST. CALORIES	PROTIEN (g)	CARBS (g)		FAT (g)
DAY	DATE	EXERCISE				BODY WEIGHT
WATER (oz)	FIBER (g)	EST. CALORIES	PROTIEN (g)	CARBS (g)		FAT (g)
DAY	DATE	EXERCISE				BODY WEIGHT
WATER (oz)	FIBER (g)	EST. CALORIES	PROTIEN (g)	CARBS (g)		FAT (g)
DAY	DATE	EXERCISE				BODY WEIGHT
WATER (oz)	FIBER (g)	EST. CALORIES	PROTIEN (g)	CARBS (g)		FAT (g)
DAY	DATE	EXERCISE				BODY WEIGHT
WATER (oz)	FIBER (g)	EST. CALORIES	PROTIEN (g)	CARBS (g)		FAT (g)
DAY	DATE	EXERCISE				BODY WEIGHT
WATER (oz)	FIBER (g)	EST. CALORIES	PROTIEN (g)	CARBS (g)		FAT (g)
DAY	DATE	EXERCISE				BODY WEIGHT
WATER (oz)	FIBER (g)	EST. CALORIES	PROTIEN (g)	CARBS (g)		FAT (g)

COMMENTS / JOURNAL / ACTION ITEMS:

_____

_____

_____

_____

_____

www.ybyl.com

SECTION 5: APPENDIX

Your Body, Your Life™

YBYL - Food Pyramid:

Caloric food volume and food combinations are important, as is the number of daily meals and snacks and total daily caloric expenditure. Negative food reactions occur most often with sugar, dairy products, wheat, peanuts, soy, wheat, corn, sodium and other additives and preservatives.

CONSUME RARELY:

SUGAR (FRUCTOSE IS BEST):
Sugar drinks, refined fruit and vegetable juices,
fruit yogurt, candy, cookies, cakes,
pies and other sugar products, ketchup, baked beans

REFINED-HIGH GLYCEMIC CARBS:
Junk food, chips, crackers, high-carb nutrition bars;
low-fiber bread, bagels and tortillas;
low-fiber breakfast cereals, pasta and rice

EXCESSIVE SATURATED FAT AND TRANS-FATTY ACIDS:
Fried foods, fatty meats, gravy and other creamy sauces,
junk food, some margarines, regular peanut butter and
vegetable oils containing trans-fatty acids

WHOLE FAT DAIRY PRODUCTS:
Whole-fat cheese, cottage cheese,
creamy salad dressings, sour cream and milk

EXCESSIVE SODIUM, ADDITIVES AND PRESERVATIVES:
Table salt, high-sodium foods and condiments

CONSUME IN MODERATION:

LOW-FIBER VEGETABLES AND FRUITS:
Peas, corn, potatoes, beets, yams, bananas, melons, grapes

MEDIUM-GLYCEMIC CARBS:
Fresh-squeezed fruit juices,
breads and cereals with at least 1g of fiber for every 5g of carb;
high-fiber, firm pasta, brown rice, oatmeal (slow-cooked)

SUPER FATS:
fish, olive, almond and peanut oils, avocadoes, olives,
low-sodium nuts and seeds, <u>natural</u> peanut or soy nut butter, almond butter, tahini

LOW-FAT DAIRY OR SOY PRODUCTS:
soymilk, soy cheese, etc.; plain/vanilla yogurt, 2 percent dairy products,
assuming no allergies or food sensitivities to dairy

OTHER:
Diet soft drinks, alcohol,
low-sodium frozen and canned foods,
egg yolks, aspartame, saccharin

CONSUME LIBERALLY:

SUPER FLUIDS:
Water, green/unsweetened tea, fresh squeezed vegetable juices

SUPER DIETARY SUPPLEMENTS:
Soluble fiber supplements, pure oat/wheat bran, sugar-free Metamucil,
high-quality multiple vitamin-mineral supplements,
additional antioxidants and minerals

SUPER FRUITS:
Strawberries, apples, peaches, pears, plums, grapefruit,
cherries, berries, oranges, lemons, limes

SUPER VEGGIES:
Spinach, greens, romaine lettuce, cucumbers, broccoli, celery, carrots,
cauliflower, cabbage, asparagus, green beans, snow peas, squash,
zucchini, sprouts, peppers, onions, mushrooms, radishes, tomatoes;
(don't overcook or use much salt, if at all.)

SUPER BEANS, LENTILS AND LEGUMES:
High-fiber/low-sodium beans
(e.g. lentils, soy, kidney, black, Great Northern, lima, navy, pinto,
garbanzo/chickpeas and blackeyed peas),
low-sodium veggie burgers

SUPER PROTEIN:
Lean meats, fish, soy products, protein shakes and bars,
egg whites, tofu, low-fat cottage cheese

SECTION 5: APPENDIX

Your Body, Your Life™

YBYL - Two-Day Detox Eating Plan

Please follow this Two-Day Plan to periodically cleanse and detoxify your body. It's a good preparatory plan if you're about to begin the YBYL Program and also good to follow monthly or on an as-needed basis, particularly on weekends. Your plan is based on your current weight.

BENEFITS:

cellular cleansing, toxin elimination, de-bloating, improved functional integrity of digestive system (gastro-intestinal tract), strengthening of immune system and improved function in the urinary, liver, respiratory, lymphatic and dermal (skin) systems.

GROCERY LIST:

soluble fiber supplement, e.g. sugar-free Metamucil, capsule or liquid multiple vitamin-mineral supplement, whey/soy protein powder or pre-made protein shakes, fresh-squeezed fruit juice, fruit, veggies, fish or canned tuna and chicken breast.

ACTIVITIES:

20 to 30 minutes of moderate aerobic exercise each day (optional); hatha yoga, stretching, deep breathing and massage, saunas, steam rooms and hot baths with Epsom salts. Keep stress low. After completing this program, ease back into your YBYL Eating Plan and reduce or completely eliminate non-nutritious foods.

DAY ONE:

	Under 140 lbs.	140-180 lbs.	180+ lbs.
Breakfast	Protein shake - 20 g	Protein shake - 25 g	Protein shake - 30 g
Mid a.m. Snack	Juice - 6 oz	Juice - 8 oz	Juice - 12 oz
Lunch	Protein shake - 20 g	Protein shake - 25 g	Protein shake - 30 g
Mid p.m. Snack	Juice - 6 oz	Juice - 8 oz	Juice - 12 oz
Dinner	Protein shake - 20 g	Protein shake - 25 g	Protein shake - 30 g
Evening Snack	Juice - 6 oz	Juice - 8 oz	Juice - 12 oz

DAY TWO:

	Under 140 lbs.	140-180 lbs.	180+ lbs.
Breakfast	Protein shake - 20 g	Protein shake - 25 g	Protein shake - 30 g
Mid a.m. Snack	Juice - 6 oz	Juice - 8 oz	Juice - 12 oz
Lunch	Large salad with tuna/fish/chicken breast		
Mid p.m. Snack	1 serving of fruit	1.5 servings of fruit	2 servings of fruit
Dinner	4-6 oz. of fish/chicken breast and 2 servings of fibrous vegetables		
Evening Snack	Juice - 6 oz	Juice - 8 oz	Juice - 12 oz

Your Body, Your Life™   SECTION 5: APPENDIX

YBYL - Super Foods List

NUTRITIONAL SUPPLEMENTS	Amt.	Cal.	Prot	Carb	Fat	Fbr.	G. I.

- Water
- High-quality multiple vitamin-mineral supplements
- Pure wheat bran and soluble fiber supplements
- Additional antioxidants
- Additional minerals for adults

NOTE: G. I. = Glycemic Index

PROTEIN SUPPLEMENTS	Amt.	Cal.	Prot	Carb	Fat	Fbr.	G. I.
Sample Protein Powder	1 scoop	155	30 g	6 g	1 g	+ bran	low
Sample Protein Bar (lo-carb)	1 bar	200	30 g	2 g	8 g	2 g	low
Sample Protein Bar	1 bar	250	30 g	19 g	6 g	1 g	low

LEAN MEATS (low-sodium)	Amt.	Cal.	Prot	Carb	Fat	Fbr.	G. I.
Chicken/Turkey, sliced, lean	3 slices	70	10 g	2 g	2 g	0 g	low
Ham/Roast Beef, sliced, lean	3 slices	80	10 g	2 g	3 g	0 g	low
Chicken/Turkey, breast, skinless	Med	196	35 g	0 g	5 g	0 g	low
Chicken/Turkey, breast, skinless	Small	136	25 g	0 g	4 g	0 g	low
Turkey, ground, extra lean	4 oz.	160	22 g	0 g	8 g	0 g	low
Beef sirloin, ground, extra lean	4 oz.	219	30 g	0 g	9 g	0 g	low
Venison, roasted	4 oz.	168	34 g	0 g	4 g	0 g	low
Pork Tenderloin/Lamb/Veal	4 oz.	193	28 g	0 g	9 g	0 g	low
Beef, round steak, lean	4 oz.	217	33 g	0 g	8 g	0 g	low
Porterhouse / Flank Steak / Beef Brisket	4 oz.	239	35 g	0 g	11 g	0 g	low

SOY PRODUCTS   High in protein and nutritious

FISH	Amt.	Cal.	Prot	Carb	Fat	Fbr.	G. I.
Bass	4 oz.	166	27 g	0 g	5.4 g	0 g	low
Catfish	4 oz.	172	21 g	0 g	9 g	0 g	low
Halibut	4 oz.	159	30 g	0 g	3.3 g	0 g	low
Lobster or Shrimp	4 oz.	112	23 g	1.5 g	1.5 g	0 g	low
Mackerel	4 oz.	297	27 g	0 g	20 g	0 g	low
Salmon	4 oz.	234	25 g	0 g	14 g	0 g	low
Trout	4 oz.	215	30 g	0 g	10 g	0 g	low
Tuna, bluefin, grilled	4 oz.	209	34 g	0 g	7 g	0 g	low

SECTION 5: APPENDIX

FISH (continued)

	Amt.	Cal.	Prot	Carb	Fat	Fbr.	G. I.
Tuna, canned, in water	4 oz.	120	26 g	0 g	1 g	0 g	low
Oysters, raw	12 med	110	12 g	6.6 g	4 g	0 g	low
Scallops	12 lge	145	30 g	4 g	1 g	0 g	low
Tuna, canned, solid white, in oil	4 oz.	180	28 g	0 g	6 g	0 g	low

"GOOD" FATS

	Amt.	Cal.	Prot	Carb	Fat	Fbr.	G. I.
Flax seeds	1.5 tbsp	70	2.5 g	5.5 g	5 g	3 g	low
Almonds	1 oz (24)	120	4 g	3.5 g	10 g	1.5 g	low
Green Olives w/pits	10 lg.	45	0.5 g	0.5 g	5 g	1 g	low
Un-salted peanuts	20	80	3.5 g	3 g	7 g	1 g	low
Tahini	2 tbsp	100	2.5 g	1.5 g	9 g	1 g	low
Black Olives w/pits	10 med	65	0.4 g	1.7 g	9 g	1 g	low
Oils - almond, canola, flaxseed, olive	1/2 tbsp	60	0 g	0 g	7 g	0 g	low
Guacamole	1 tbsp	60	0.5 g	1 g	6 g	0 g	low
Avocado, raw	1/4	88	1 g	3 g	8 g	0 g	low
Almond Butter	1/2 oz	92	2.5 g	3 g	8 g	0 g	low
Natural/Soy Peanut Butter	1 tbsp	100	4.5 g	6 g	6 g	1 g	low

DAIRY PRODUCTS

	Amt.	Cal.	Prot	Carb	Fat	Fbr.	G. I.
Cottage cheese, low-fat, low sodium	1/2 cup	90	14 g	4 g	2.5 g	0 g	low
Cottage cheese, fat-free, low sodium	1/2 cup	70	14 g	4 g	0 g	0 g	low
Milk, soy	8 oz	100	6 g	10 g	3.5 g	0 g	low
Milk, skim	8 oz	86	8 g	12 g	0 g	0 g	low
Milk, 1%	8 oz	102	8 g	12 g	3 g	0 g	low
Egg, whole	1	80	6 g	1 g	6 g	0 g	low
Egg whites	1	16	4 g	0.3 g	0 g	0 g	low
Egg white substitute	1/4 cup	30	6 g	1 g	0 g	0 g	low
Yogurt, low-fat, plain	8 oz	139	12 g	16 g	3 g	0 g	low
Parmesan Cheese, grated	2 tsp	25	2 g	0 g	1.5 g	0 g	low
Mayonnaisse, low fat	1 tsp	50	0 g	8 g	2 g	0 g	low

VEGETABLES

	Amt.	Cal.	Prot	Carb	Fat	Fbr.	G. I.
Asparagus	4 spears	14	1.3 g	2.6 g	0 g	1.2 g	low
Broccoli, fresh	1 cup	42	4.5 g	8 g	0.5	5 g	low
Broccoli, frozen	10 oz	84	8.7 g	15 g	1 g	8.5 g	low
Cabbage / Cauliflower	1 cup	34	1.6 g	6.8 g	0 g	4.2 g	low
Celery	1 stalk	6	0.3 g	1.5 g	0 g	0.7 g	low
Cucumber	1 lge	38	2 g	8 g	0 g	2.4 g	low
Green beans	1 cup	44	2 g	10 g	0 g	4 g	low
Green Peas, dried	1/4 cup	100	9 g	24 g	0 g	9 g	low

SECTION 5: APPENDIX

VEGETABLES (continued)	Amt.	Cal.	Prot	Carb	Fat	Fbr.	G. I.
Green pepper	1 cup	26	0.8 g	6.4 g	0.2 g	1.8 g	low
Greens	1 cup	60	2 g	16 g	1 g	8 g	low
Hummus	1 oz	85	3.5 g	7.5 g	4.5 g	0 g	low
Lettuce, romaine	2 cups	16	2 g	2.8 g	0 g	2.8 g	low
Mushrooms, boiled	1 cup	42	4 g	8 g	0 g	3.4 g	low
Onion, chopped	1/2 cup	30	1 g	7 g	0 g	1.4 g	low
Radishes, sliced	1/2 cup	10	0.4 g	2 g	0.3 g	0.9 g	low
Snow peas, boiled	1/2 cup	34	2.6 g	5.6 g	0.2 g	2.2 g	low
Spinach, boiled	1 cup	42	5.4 g	6.8 g	0.4 g	4.4 g	low
Tomato, chopped	1/2 cup	19	0.8 g	4.2 g	0.3 g	1 g	low
Yellow squash	1/2 cup	25	0 g	5 g	0 g	2 g	low
Zucchini, boiled	1/2 cup	14	0.6 g	3.5 g	0.1 g	1.3 g	low

BREAD / BRAN / GRAIN	Amt.	Cal.	Prot	Carb	Fat	Fbr.	G. I.
Oat Bran or Wheat Bran	Buy this stuff; it's pure soluble fiber! Add to foods!						low
Breads	Go for high fiber, moderate carbs						med
Breakfast Cereals	Go for high fiber, moderate carbs and add bran						med
Other Cereals and Pancake Mix	Go for high fiber, moderate carbs and add bran						med
Oatmeal, slow-cooked	1/2 cup	150	5 g	27 g	3 g	+ bran	med
Pastas	Don't overcook; eat with protein-based sauce						

LEGUMES	Amt.	Cal.	Prot	Carb	Fat	Fbr.	G. I.
Soy beans	1/2 cup	127	11 g	10 g	6 g	5.4 g	low
Kidney Beans / Lentils	1/2 cup	116	9 g	20 g	0.4 g	7 g	low
Black beans / Great Northern beans	1/2 cup	96	6.5 g	17.5 g	0 g	6 g	low
Navy / Lima / Pinto / Garbanzo beans	1/2 cup	110	6 g	18 g	1.5 g	5 g	low
Black-eyed peas	1/2 cup	90	6 g	16 g	0 g	3 g	med
Vegetable Burgers (low sodium)	Go for high fiber, high protein and moderate carbs.						

SUPER FRUITS	Amt.	Cal.	Prot	Carb	Fat	Fbr.	G. I.
Cherries	1/2 cup	26	0.5 g	6.3 g	0.2 g	0.6 g	low
Plum	1	36	0.5 g	8.6 g	0.4 g	1 g	low
Grapefruit	1 med	92	1.2 g	24 g	0 g	5 g	low
Banana, unripe (green)	1 med	105	1.2 g	27 g	0.6 g	3 g	med
Strawberries	1 pint	97	2 g	22 g	1.2 g	7.4 g	low
Blackberries/Blueberries/Rasperies	1/2 cup	40	1 g	9 g	0 g	3.6 g	med
Apple / Pear	1 med	94	0.5 g	23 g	0 g	4 g	med
Applesauce, unsweetened	1/2 cup	42	0 g	14 g	0 g	0 g	med
Grapes, seedless	10 med	36	0.3 g	9 g	0.3 g	0.3 g	med
Orange	1 med	65	1.4 g	16.3 g	0 g	3.4 g	med

www.ybyl.com

SECTION 5: APPENDIX

Your Body, Your Life™

NON-SUPER (CHEAT) FOODS	Amt.	Cal.	Prot	Carb	Fat	Fbr.	G. I.
Beer, regular	12 oz.	150	1 g	13 g	0 g	0 g	med
Beer, light	12 oz.	95	1 g	4 g	0 g	0 g	low
Red or white wine	7 oz.	175	0 g	8.4 g	0 g	0 g	med
Gin/run/vodka/whiskey (80 proof)	1 shot	95	0 g	0 g	0 g	0 g	low
Soft drink, regular	12 oz.	150	0 g	41 g	0 g	0 g	high
Orange Juice, refined	12 oz.	158	1.5 g	37.5 g	1 g	0 g	high
Yogurt, fruit flavored	8 oz.	230	10 g	43 g	2 g	0 g	high
Cheese	1 slice	105	6 g	1 g	9 g	0 g	low
Ice Cream, regular	1 cup	270	5 g	32 g	14 g	0 g	high
Salad Dressing, ranch	3 tbs	255	1 g	3 g	27 g	0 g	low
Bread, whole wheat	1 slice	70	3 g	13 g	1 g	2 g	high
Bagel	1	200	7 g	38 g	2 g	0 g	high
Biscuit	1	100	2 g	13 g	5 g	0 g	high
Croissant	1	235	5 g	27 g	12 g	0 g	high
Cheesecake	1 slice	280	5 g	26 g	18 g	0 g	high
Chocolate Chip Cookies	4	180	2 g	28 g	9 g	0 g	high
Rice, white	1 cup	225	4 g	50 g	1 g	0 g	high
Pasta, low-fiber	1 cup	190	7 g	39 g	1 g	0 g	high
Enchilada	1	235	20 g	24 g	16 g	2 g	med
Sugar	1 tbs	45	0 g	12 g	0 g	0 g	high
Baked Potato, 8 oz	1	220	5 g	51 g	1 g	0 g	high
Potato Chips	20	210	2 g	20 g	14 g	0 g	high
Catsup	3 tbs	45	tr	15 g	0 g	0 g	high

Your Body, Your Life™

YBYL - Super Foods Grocery List

LEAN MEATS

Chicken / Turkey sliced, lean, low-sodium
Chicken / Turkey breast, skinless
Ham / Roast Beef sliced, lean, low-sodium
Turkey - ground extra lean
Venison
Pork Tenderloin / Lamb / Veal
Beef - sirloin ground, extra lean
Beef - round steak lean
Beef - porterhouse / flank steak / beef brisket

FISH

Bass, Catfish, Trout
Halibut
Lobster or Shrimp
Salmon, Mackerel, Tuna
Tuna, canned, solid white, in oil
Tuna, canned, in water
Oysters, Scallops

DAIRY PRODUCTS

Cottage cheese, low-fat
Cottage cheese, fat-free
Milk, soy
Milk, skim
Milk, 1%
Egg, whole
Egg whites
Egg white substitute
Yogurt, low-fat, plain
Parmesan Cheese, grated
Mayonaisse, low fat

DRINKS / JUICES

Crystal Light & Tang, sugar-free
Fresh-squeezed veggie and fruit juice
Green Tea (antioxidant qualities)

www.ybyl.com

SECTION 5: APPENDIX

OTHER GOOD FATS (Consume moderately due to high calorie content)

Tahini
Flax seeds
Almonds
Almond, Canola, Flax seed, Olive Oils
Black Olives w/pits
Green Olives w/pits
Guacamole
Un-salted peanuts
Almond Butter
Natural Peanut Butter or Soy Nut Butter

BREAD / BRAN / GRAIN

Oat Bran or Wheat Bran
Orowheat Light, 100% whole wheat
Roman Meal Oat Bran Light
El Galindo Whole wheat tortillas, fat-free
Kellogg's Bran Buds/All-bran extra fiber
Cereals with at least 1g of fiber per 5g of carbs
Oatmeal, slow-cooked
Hodgson Mill whole wheat pastas
Add wheat bran to increase fiber content

LEGUMES

Soy beans
Kidney Beans / Lentils
Black beans / Great Northern beans
Lima beans
Beans (Navy, Pinto, Garbanzo)
Black-eyed peas
Soy Products, Tofu
Vegetable Burgers (low sodium)

MISCELLANEOUS

Salsa, lime juice, lemon juice
Fructose or Stevia (sweetener)
Soluble Fiber Supplements
High-quality multiple vitamin-mineral supplements
Additional anti-oxidant and mineral supplements

SECTION 5: APPENDIX

VEGETABLES (Rinse canned vegetables if high in sodium)

Asparagus
Broccoli, fresh
Broccoli, frozen
Cabbage / Cauliflower
Celery
Cucumber
Green beans
Green pepper
Green peas, dried
Greens
Hummus
Lettuce, romaine
Mushrooms
Onions
Radishes
Snow peas
Spinach
Tomato
Yellow squash
Zucchini

SUPER FRUITS

Apple / Pear
Applesauce, unsweetened
Banana, unripe (green)
Blackberries/Blueberries/Rasperies
Cherries
Grapefruits, Oranges
Plum
Strawberries
Grapes, seedless

NOTES:
- Go grocery shopping on a full stomach!
- Search for low-sodium products!
- Search for high fiber products!
- Keep non-nutritious foods out of your home!

www.ybyl.com

SECTION 5: APPENDIX

YBYL Daily Eating Plan - Calories
(40%-protein, 30%-carb, 30%-fat)

DAILY CALORIES	BREAKFAST CALORIES	SNACK 1 CALORIES	LUNCH CALORIES	SNACK 2 CALORIES	DINNER CALORIES
1,000	250	125	250	125	250
1,100	275	138	275	138	275
1,200	300	150	300	150	300
1,300	325	163	325	163	325
1,400	350	175	350	175	350
1,500	375	188	375	188	375
1,600	400	200	400	200	400
1,700	425	213	425	213	425
1,800	450	225	450	225	450
1,900	475	238	475	238	475
2,000	500	250	500	250	500
2,100	525	263	525	263	525
2,200	550	275	550	275	550
2,300	575	288	575	288	575
2,400	600	300	600	300	600
2,500	625	313	625	313	625

YBYL Daily Eating Plan - Amounts
(40%-protein, 30%-carb, 30%-fat)

DAILY CALORIES	DAILY PROTEIN	DAILY CARBS	DAILY FAT	MEAL PROTEIN	MEAL CARBS	MEAL FAT	SNACK PROTEIN	SNACK CARBS	SNACK FAT
1,000	100 g	75 g	33 g	25 g	19 g	8 g	13 g	9 g	4 g
1,100	110 g	83 g	37 g	28 g	21 g	9 g	14 g	10 g	5 g
1,200	120 g	90 g	40 g	30 g	23 g	10 g	15 g	11 g	5 g
1,300	130 g	98 g	43 g	33 g	24 g	11 g	16 g	12 g	5 g
1,400	140 g	105 g	47 g	35 g	26 g	12 g	18 g	13 g	6 g
1,500	150 g	113 g	50 g	38 g	28 g	13 g	19 g	14 g	6 g
1,600	160 g	120 g	53 g	40 g	30 g	13 g	20 g	15 g	7 g
1,700	170 g	128 g	57 g	43 g	32 g	14 g	21 g	16 g	7 g
1,800	180 g	135 g	60 g	45 g	34 g	15 g	23 g	17 g	8 g
1,900	190 g	143 g	63 g	48 g	36 g	16 g	24 g	18 g	8 g
2,000	200 g	150 g	67 g	50 g	38 g	17 g	25 g	19 g	8 g
2,100	210 g	158 g	70 g	53 g	39 g	18 g	26 g	20 g	9 g
2,200	220 g	165 g	73 g	55 g	41 g	18 g	28 g	21 g	9 g
2,300	230 g	173 g	77 g	58 g	43 g	19 g	29 g	22 g	10 g
2,400	240 g	180 g	80 g	60 g	45 g	20 g	30 g	23 g	10 g
2,500	250 g	188 g	83 g	63 g	47 g	21 g	31 g	23 g	10 g

SECTION 5: APPENDIX

Your Body, Your Life™

1200 Calories, Meal & Snack Plan
(40%-protein, 30%-carb, 30%-fat)

MEALS: 300 Calories / SNACKS: half these quantities

PROTEIN

(30 g)	Amount
Lean meat	4 oz
Fish	4 oz
Chicken breast	med
Lean, low-salt lunch meat	3-5 slices
Can tuna, in water (rinse)	4 oz

(30 g)	Amount
Low-fat cottage cheese	1 cup
Egg whites	7
Protein drinks/bars	check
Low-sodium soy burgers	check
Tofu / soy products	check

CARBOHYDRATES

(23 g)	Amount
High-fiber vegetables/salads	unlimited
Corn/peas/carrots	0.5 cup
Baked potato, med	half
Bread, whole wheat	check
Bagel	half
Pasta	0.75 cup
Rice	0.5 cup
Milk, soy/skim or 1%	16 oz
Fresh-squeezed juices	8 oz
Yogurt, low-fat, plain/vanilla	8 oz

(23 g)	Amount
Yogurt, fruit flavored	4 oz
Beans/lentils/legumes	1 cup
Banana/apple/pear/orange	1
Grapefruit	1
Strawberries/Blueberries	1 cup
Grapes	30
Plums	3
Oat meal, slow-cooked	0.5 cup
High-fiber cereals	check
Protein drinks/bars	check

FAT

(10 g)	Amount
Fat from lean meat & fish	4 oz
Creamy salad dressing	1 TBS
Cheese, sliced	1 slice
Guacamole	2 TBS
Avocado	0.25
Nuts, unsalted	15-20
Egg yolks	2

(10 g)	Amount
Natural / soy-nut peanut butter	1 TBS
Almond butter	1 TBS
Olive/canola Oil	0.5 TBS
Peanut/almond/flaxseed Oil	0.5 TBS
Flaxseeds, whole	3 TBS
Olives (rinse)	10

Your Body, Your Life™

SECTION 5: APPENDIX

1500 Calories, Meal & Snack Plan
[40%-protein, 30%-carb, 30%-fat]

MEALS: 375 Calories / SNACKS: half these quantities

PROTEIN

(38 g)	Amount	(38 g)	Amount
Lean meat	5 oz	Low-fat cottage cheese	1.25 cups
Fish	5 oz	Egg whites	8.5
Chicken breast	med	Protein drinks/bars	check
Lean, low-salt lunch meat	4-6 slices	Low-sodium soy burgers	check
Can tuna, in water (rinse)	5 oz	Tofu/soy products	check

CARBOHYDRATES

(28 g)	Amount	(28 g)	Amount
High-fiber vegetables/salads	unlimited	Yogurt, fruit flavored	5 oz
Corn/peas/carrots	0.75 cup	Beans/lentils/legumes	1.25 cups
Baked potato, med	half	Banana/apple/pear/orange	1.25
Bread, whole wheat	check	Grapefruit	1.25
Bagel	half	Strawberries/Blueberries	1.25 cups
Pasta	1 cup	Grapes	30
Rice	0.5 cup	Plums	4
Milk, soy/skim or 1%	20 oz	Oat meal, slow-cooked	0.5 cup
Fresh-squeezed juices	10 oz	High-fiber cereals	check
Yogurt, low-fat, plain/vanilla	10 oz	Protein drinks/bars	check

FAT

(13 g)	Amount	(13 g)	Amount
Fat from lean meat & fish	5 oz	Natural / soy-nut peanut butter	1.25 TBS
Creamy salad dressing	1 TBS	Almond butter	1.25 TBS
Cheese, sliced	1 slice	Olive/canola Oil	0.5 TBS
Guacamole	2 TBS	Peanut/almond/flaxseed Oil	0.5 TBS
Avocado	0.33	Flaxseeds, whole	3 TBS
Nuts, unsalted	18-22	Olives (rinse)	12
Egg yolks	2	Low-carb Protein bars	check

www.ybyl.com

SECTION 5: APPENDIX

1800 Calories, Meal & Snack Plan
[40%-protein, 30%-carb, 30%-fat]

MEALS: 450 Calories / SNACKS: half these quantities

PROTEIN

(45 g)	Amount
Lean meat	6 oz
Fish	6 oz
Chicken breast	large
Lean, low-salt lunch meat	5-7 slices
Can tuna, in water (rinse)	6 oz

(45 g)	Amount
Low-fat cottage cheese	1.5 cups
Egg whites	10
Protein drinks/bars	check
Low-sodium soy burgers	check
Tofu/soy products	check

CARBOHYDRATES

(34 g)	Amount
High-fiber vegetables/salads	unlimited
Corn/peas/carrots	1 cup
Baked potato, med	half
Bread, whole wheat	check
Bagel	0.75
Pasta	1.25 cups
Rice	0.75 cup
Milk, soy/skim or 1%	24 oz
Fresh-squeezed juices	12 oz
Yogurt, low-fat, plain/vanilla	12 oz

(34 g)	Amount
Yogurt, fruit flavored	6 oz
Beans/lentils/legumes	1.5 cups
Banana/apple/pear/orange	1.5
Grapefruit	1.5
Strawberries/Blueberries	1.5 cups
Grapes	45
Plums	5
Oat meal, slow-cooked	0.75 cup
High-fiber cereals	check
Protein drinks/bars	check

FAT

(15 g)	Amount
Fat from lean meat & fish	6 oz
Creamy salad dressing	1.5 TBS
Cheese, sliced	1.5 slices
Guacamole	3 TBS
Avocado	0.5
Nuts, unsalted	20-25
Egg yolks	3

(15 g)	Amount
Natural / soy-nut peanut butter	1.5 TBS
Almond butter	1.5 TBS
Olive/canola Oil	0.75 TBS
Peanut/almond/flaxseed Oil	0.75 TBS
Flaxseeds, whole	4.5 TBS
Olives (rinse)	15
Low-carb Protein bars	check

SECTION 5: APPENDIX

2100 Calories, Meal & Snack Plan
[40%-protein, 30%-carb, 30%-fat]

MEALS: 525 Calories / SNACKS: half these quantities

PROTEIN

(53 g)	Amount	(53 g)	Amount
Lean meat	7 oz	Low-fat cottage cheese	1.5 cups
Fish	7 oz	Egg whites	12
Chicken breast	large	Protein drinks/bars	check
Lean, low-salt lunch meat	6-8 slices	Low-sodium soy burgers	check
Can tuna, in water (rinse)	7 oz	Tofu/soy products	check

CARBOHYDRATES

(39 g)	Amount	(39 g)	Amount
High-fiber vegetables/salads	unlimited	Yogurt, fruit flavored	8 oz
Corn/peas/carrots	1.25 cups	Beans/lentils/legumes	1.75 cups
Baked potato, med	half	Banana/apple/pear/orange	1.75
Bread, whole wheat	check	Grapefruit	1.75
Bagel	0.75	Strawberries/Blueberries	1.75 cups
Pasta	1.25 cups	Grapes	50
Rice	1 cup	Plums	6
Milk, soy/skim or 1%	24 oz	Oat meal, slow-cooked	1 cup
Fresh-squeezed juices	12 oz	High-fiber cereals	check
Yogurt, low-fat, plain/vanilla	12 oz	Protein drinks/bars	check

FAT

(18 g)	Amount	(18 g)	Amount
Fat from lean meat & fish	7 oz	Natural / soy-nut peanut butter	1.75 TBS
Creamy salad dressing	1.75 TBS	Almond butter	1.75 TBS
Cheese, sliced	1.75 slices	Olive/canola Oil	1 TBS
Guacamole	3.5 TBS	Peanut/almond/flaxseed Oil	1 TBS
Avocado	0.6	Flaxseeds, whole	5 TBS
Nuts, unsalted	20-25	Olives (rinse)	18
Egg yolks	3.5	Low-carb Protein bars	check

www.ybyl.com

SECTION 5: APPENDIX

YBYL Daily Eating Plan - Calories
(40%-protein, 40%-carb, 20%-fat)

DAILY CALORIES	BREAKFAST CALORIES	SNACK 1 CALORIES	LUNCH CALORIES	SNACK 2 CALORIES	DINNER CALORIES
1,000	250	125	250	125	250
1,100	275	138	275	138	275
1,200	300	150	300	150	300
1,300	325	163	325	163	325
1,400	350	175	350	175	350
1,500	375	188	375	188	375
1,600	400	200	400	200	400
1,700	425	213	425	213	425
1,800	450	225	450	225	450
1,900	475	238	475	238	475
2,000	500	250	500	250	500
2,100	525	263	525	263	525
2,200	550	275	550	275	550
2,300	575	288	575	288	575
2,400	600	300	600	300	600
2,500	625	313	625	313	625

SECTION 5: APPENDIX

YBYL Daily Eating Plan - Amounts
[40%-protein, 40%-carb, 20%-fat]

DAILY CALORIES	DAILY PROTEIN	DAILY CARBS	DAILY FAT	MEAL PROTEIN	MEAL CARBS	MEAL FAT	SNACK PROTEIN	SNACK CARBS	SNACK FAT
1,000	100 g	100 g	22 g	25 g	25 g	6 g	13 g	13 g	3 g
1,100	110 g	110 g	24 g	28 g	28 g	6 g	14 g	14 g	3 g
1,200	120 g	120 g	27 g	30 g	30 g	7 g	15 g	15 g	3 g
1,300	130 g	130 g	29 g	33 g	33 g	7 g	16 g	16 g	4 g
1,400	140 g	140 g	31 g	35 g	35 g	8 g	18 g	18 g	4 g
1,500	150 g	150 g	33 g	38 g	38 g	8 g	19 g	19 g	4 g
1,600	160 g	160 g	36 g	40 g	40 g	9 g	20 g	20 g	4 g
1,700	170 g	170 g	38 g	43 g	43 g	9 g	21 g	21 g	5 g
1,800	180 g	180 g	40 g	45 g	45 g	10 g	23 g	23 g	5 g
1,900	190 g	190 g	42 g	48 g	48 g	11 g	24 g	24 g	5 g
2,000	200 g	200 g	44 g	50 g	50 g	11 g	25 g	25 g	6 g
2,100	210 g	210 g	47 g	53 g	53 g	12 g	26 g	26 g	6 g
2,200	220 g	220 g	49 g	55 g	55 g	12 g	28 g	28 g	6 g
2,300	230 g	230 g	51 g	58 g	58 g	13 g	29 g	29 g	6 g
2,400	240 g	240 g	53 g	60 g	60 g	13 g	30 g	30 g	7 g
2,500	250 g	250 g	56 g	63 g	63 g	14 g	31 g	31 g	7 g

www.ybyl.com

SECTION 5: APPENDIX

Your Body, Your Life™

1200 Calories, Meal & Snack Plan
(40%-protein, 40%-carb, 20%-fat)

MEALS: 300 Calories / SNACKS: half these quantities

PROTEIN

(30 g)	Amount
Lean meat	4 oz
Fish	4 oz
Chicken breast	med
Lean, low-salt lunch meat	3-5 slices
Can tuna, in water (rinse)	4 oz

(30 g)	Amount
Low-fat cottage cheese	1 cup
Egg whites	7
Protein drinks/bars	check
Low-sodium soy burgers	check
Tofu/soy products	check

CARBOHYDRATES

(30 g)	Amount
High-fiber vegetables/salads	unlimited
Corn/peas/carrots	0.75 cup
Baked potato, med	half
Bread, whole wheat	check
Bagel	half
Pasta	1 cup
Rice	0.5 cup
Milk, soy/skim or 1%	20 oz
Fresh-squeezed juices	10 oz
Yogurt, low-fat, plain/vanilla	10 oz

(30 g)	Amount
Yogurt, fruit flavored	5 oz
Beans/lentils/legumes	1.25 cups
Banana/apple/pear/orange	1.25
Grapefruit	1.25
Strawberries/Blueberries	1.25 cups
Grapes	30
Plums	4
Oat meal, slow-cooked	0.5 cup
High-fiber cereals	check
Protein drinks/bars	check

FAT

(7 g)	Amount
Fat from lean meat & fish	2.5 oz
Creamy salad dressing	0.5 TBS
Cheese, sliced	0.75 slice
Guacamole	1.5 TBS
Avocado	0.25
Nuts, unsalted	12-15
Egg yolks	2

(7 g)	Amount
Natural / soy-nut peanut butter	0.75 TBS
Almond butter	0.75 TBS
Olive/canola Oil	0.5 TBS
Peanut/almond/flaxseed Oil	0.5 TBS
Flaxseeds, whole	2.5 TBS
Olives (rinse)	7

www.ybyl.com

1500 Calories, Meal & Snack Plan
[40%-protein, 40%-carb, 20%-fat]

MEALS: 375 Calories / SNACKS: half these quantities

PROTEIN

(38 g)	Amount	(38 g)	Amount
Lean meat	5 oz	Low-fat cottage cheese	1.25 cups
Fish	5 oz	Egg whites	8.5
Chicken breast	med	Protein drinks/bars	check
Lean, low-salt lunch meat	4-6 slices	Low-sodium soy burgers	check
Can tuna, in water (rinse)	5 oz	Tofu/soy products	check

CARBOHYDRATES

(38 g)	Amount	(38 g)	Amount
High-fiber vegetables/salads	unlimited	Yogurt, fruit flavored	8 oz
Corn/peas/carrots	1.25 cups	Beans/lentils/legumes	1.75 cups
Baked potato, med	half	Banana/apple/pear/orange	1.75
Bread, whole wheat	check	Grapefruit	1.75
Bagel	0.75	Strawberries/Blueberries	1.75 cups
Pasta	1.25 cups	Grapes	50
Rice	1 cup	Plums	6
Milk, soy/skim or 1%	24 oz	Oat meal, slow-cooked	1 cup
Fresh-squeezed juices	12 oz	High-fiber cereals	check
Yogurt, low-fat, plain/vanilla	12 oz	Protein drinks/bars	check

FAT

(8 g)	Amount	(8 g)	Amount
Fat from lean meat & fish	2.5 oz	Natural / soy-nut peanut butter	0.75 TBS
Creamy salad dressing	0.5 TBS	Almond butter	0.75 TBS
Cheese, sliced	0.75 slice	Olive/canola Oil	0.5 TBS
Guacamole	1.5 TBS	Peanut/almond/flaxseed Oil	0.5 TBS
Avocado	0.25	Flaxseeds, whole	2.5 TBS
Nuts, unsalted	12-15	Olives (rinse)	7
Egg yolks	2	Low-carb Protein bars	check

SECTION 5: APPENDIX

Your Body, Your Life™

1800 Calories, Meal & Snack Plan
[40%-protein, 40%-carb, 20%-fat]

MEALS: 450 Calories / SNACKS: half these quantities

PROTEIN

(45 g)	Amount
Lean meat	6 oz
Fish	6 oz
Chicken breast	large
Lean, low-salt lunch meat	5-7 slices
Can tuna, in water (rinse)	6 oz

(45 g)	Amount
Low-fat cottage cheese	1.5 cups
Egg whites	10
Protein drinks/bars	check
Low-sodium soy burgers	check
Tofu/soy products	check

CARBOHYDRATES

(45 g)	Amount
High-fiber vegetables/salads	unlimited
Corn/peas/carrots	1 cup
Baked potato, med	1
Bread, whole wheat	check
Bagel	1
Pasta	1.5 cups
Rice	1 cup
Milk, soy/skim or 1%	32 oz
Fresh-squeezed juices	16 oz
Yogurt, low-fat, plain/vanilla	16 oz

(45 g)	Amount
Yogurt, fruit flavored	8 oz
Beans/lentils/legumes	2 cups
Banana/apple/pear/orange	2
Grapefruit	2
Strawberries/Blueberries	2 cups
Grapes	60
Plums	6
Oat meal, slow-cooked	1 cup
High-fiber cereals	check
Protein drinks/bars	check

FAT

(10 g)	Amount
Fat from lean meat & fish	4 oz
Creamy salad dressing	1 TBS
Cheese, sliced	1 slice
Guacamole	2 TBS
Avocado	0.25
Nuts, unsalted	15-20
Egg yolks	2

(10 g)	Amount
Natural / soy-nut peanut butter	1 TBS
Almond butter	1 TBS
Olive/canola Oil	0.5 TBS
Peanut/almond/flaxseed Oil	0.5 TBS
Flaxseeds, whole	3 TBS
Olives (rinse)	10
Low-carb Protein bars	check

Your Body, Your Life™

SECTION 5: APPENDIX

2100 Calories, Meal & Snack Plan
[40%-protein, 40%-carb, 20%-fat]

MEALS: 525 Calories / SNACKS: half these quantities

PROTEIN

(53 g)	Amount
Lean meat	7 oz
Fish	7 oz
Chicken breast	large
Lean, low-salt lunch meat	6-8 slices
Can tuna, in water (rinse)	6 oz

(53 g)	Amount
Low-fat cottage cheese	1.5 cups
Egg whites	12
Protein drinks/bars	check
Low-sodium soy burgers	check
Tofu/soy products	check

CARBOHYDRATES

(53 g)	Amount
High-fiber vegetables/salads	unlimited
Corn/peas/carrots	1.25 cups
Baked potato,	med
Bread, whole wheat	check
Bagel	1
Pasta	1.75 cups
Rice	1.25 cups
Milk, soy/skim or 1%	40 oz
Fresh-squeezed juices	20 oz
Yogurt, low-fat, plain/vanilla	20 oz

(53 g)	Amount
Yogurt, fruit flavored	10 oz
Beans/lentils/legumes	2.5 cups
Banana/apple/pear/orange	2.5
Grapefruit	2.5
Strawberries/Blueberries	2.25 cups
Grapes	70
Plums	8
Oat meal, slow-cooked	1.25 cups
High-fiber cereals	check
Protein drinks/bars	check

FAT

(12 g)	Amount
Fat from lean meat & fish	5 oz
Creamy salad dressing	1.25 TBS
Cheese, sliced	1.25 slices
Guacamole	2.25 TBS
Avocado	0.33
Nuts, unsalted	20
Egg yolks	2.5

(12 g)	Amount
Natural / soy-nut peanut butter	1.25 TBS
Almond butter	1.25 TBS
Olive/canola Oil	0.75 TBS
Peanut/almond/flaxseed Oil	0.75 TBS
Flaxseeds, whole	3.5 TBS
Olives (rinse)	12
Low-carb Protein bars	check

www.ybyl.com

SECTION 5: APPENDIX

YBYL Daily Eating Plan - Calories
[30%-protein, 50%-carb, 20%-fat]

DAILY CALORIES	BREAKFAST CALORIES	SNACK 1 CALORIES	LUNCH CALORIES	SNACK 2 CALORIES	DINNER CALORIES
1,000	250	125	250	125	250
1,100	275	138	275	138	275
1,200	300	150	300	150	300
1,300	325	163	325	163	325
1,400	350	175	350	175	350
1,500	375	188	375	188	375
1,600	400	200	400	200	400
1,700	425	213	425	213	425
1,800	450	225	450	225	450
1,900	475	238	475	238	475
2,000	500	250	500	250	500
2,100	525	263	525	263	525
2,200	550	275	550	275	550
2,300	575	288	575	288	575
2,400	600	300	600	300	600
2,500	625	313	625	313	625

YBYL Daily Eating Plan - Amounts
(30%-protein, 50%-carb, 20%-fat)

DAILY CALORIES	DAILY PROTEIN	DAILY CARBS	DAILY FAT	MEAL PROTEIN	MEAL CARBS	MEAL FAT	SNACK PROTEIN	SNACK CARBS	SNACK FAT
1,000	75 g	125 g	22 g	19 g	31 g	6 g	9 g	16 g	3 g
1,100	83 g	138 g	24 g	21 g	34 g	6 g	10 g	17 g	3 g
1,200	90 g	150 g	27 g	23 g	38 g	7 g	11 g	19 g	3 g
1,300	98 g	163 g	29 g	24 g	41 g	7 g	12 g	20 g	4 g
1,400	105 g	175 g	31 g	26 g	44 g	8 g	13 g	22 g	4 g
1,500	113 g	188 g	33 g	28 g	47 g	8 g	14 g	23 g	4 g
1,600	120 g	200 g	36 g	30 g	50 g	9 g	15 g	25 g	4 g
1,700	128 g	213 g	38 g	32 g	53 g	9 g	16 g	27 g	5 g
1,800	135 g	225 g	40 g	34 g	56 g	10 g	17 g	28 g	5 g
1,900	143 g	238 g	42 g	36 g	59 g	11 g	18 g	30 g	5 g
2,000	150 g	250 g	44 g	38 g	63 g	11 g	19 g	31 g	6 g
2,100	158 g	263 g	47 g	39 g	66 g	12 g	20 g	33 g	6 g
2,200	165 g	275 g	49 g	41 g	69 g	12 g	21 g	34 g	6 g
2,300	173 g	288 g	51 g	43 g	72 g	13 g	22 g	36 g	6 g
2,400	180 g	300 g	53 g	45 g	75 g	13 g	23 g	38 g	7 g
2,500	188 g	313 g	56 g	47 g	78 g	14 g	23 g	39 g	7 g

SECTION 5: APPENDIX

Your Body, Your Life™

1200 Calories, Meal & Snack Plan
(30%-protein, 50%-carb, 20%-fat)

MEALS: 300 Calories / SNACKS: half these quantities

PROTEIN

(23 g)	Amount	(23 g)	Amount
Lean meat	3 oz	Low-fat cottage cheese	0.75 cups
Fish	3 oz	Egg whites	5
Chicken breast	small	Protein drinks/bars	check
Lean, low-salt lunch meat	2-3 slices	Low-sodium soy burgers	check
Can tuna, in water (rinse)	3 oz	Tofu/soy products	check

CARBOHYDRATES

(38 g)	Amount	(38 g)	Amount
High-fiber vegetables/salads	unlimited	Yogurt, fruit flavored	8 oz
Corn/peas/carrots	1.25 cups	Beans/lentils/legumes	1.75 cups
Baked potato, med	half	Banana/apple/pear/orange	1.75
Bread, whole wheat	check	Grapefruit	1.75
Bagel	0.75	Strawberries/Blueberries	1.75 cups
Pasta	1.25 cups	Grapes	50
Rice	1 cup	Plums	6
Milk, soy/skim or 1%	24 oz	Oat meal, slow-cooked	1 cup
Fresh-squeezed juices	12 oz	High-fiber cereals	check
Yogurt, low-fat, plain/vanilla	12 oz	Protein drinks/bars	check

FAT

(7 g)	Amount	(7 g)	Amount
Fat from lean meat & fish	2.5 oz	Natural / soy-nut peanut butter	0.75 TBS
Creamy salad dressing	0.5 TBS	Almond butter	0.75 TBS
Cheese, sliced	0.75 slice	Olive/canola Oil	0.5 TBS
Guacamole	1.5 TBS	Peanut/almond/flaxseed Oil	0.5 TBS
Avocado	0.25	Flaxseeds, whole	2.5 TBS
Nuts, unsalted	12-15	Olives (rinse)	7
Egg yolks	2		

www.ybyl.com

Your Body, Your Life™

SECTION 5: APPENDIX

1500 Calories, Meal & Snack Plan
[30%-protein, 50%-carb, 20%-fat]

MEALS: 375 Calories / SNACKS: half these quantities

PROTEIN

(28 g)	Amount
Lean meat	4 oz
Fish	4 oz
Chicken breast	med
Lean, low-salt lunch meat	3-5 slices
Can tuna, in water (rinse)	4 oz

(28 g)	Amount
Low-fat cottage cheese	1 cup
Egg whites	7
Protein drinks/bars	check
Low-sodium soy burgers	check
Tofu / soy products	check

CARBOHYDRATES

(47 g)	Amount
High-fiber vegetables/salads	unlimited
Corn/peas/carrots	1 cup
Baked potato, med	1
Bread, whole wheat	check
Bagel	1
Pasta	1:5 cups
Rice	1 cup
Milk, soy/skim or 1%	32 oz
Fresh-squeezed juices	16 oz
Yogurt, low-fat, plain/vanilla	16 oz

(47 g)	Amount
Yogurt, fruit flavored	8 oz
Beans/lentils/legumes	2 cups
Banana/apple/pear/orange	2
Grapefruit	2
Strawberries/Blueberries	2 cups
Grapes	60
Plums	6
Oat meal, slow-cooked	1 cup
High-fiber cereals	check
Protein drinks/bars	check

FAT

(8 g)	Amount
Fat from lean meat & fish	2.5 oz
Creamy salad dressing	0.5 TBS
Cheese, sliced	0.75 slice
Guacamole	1.5 TBS
Avocado	0.25
Nuts, unsalted	12-15
Egg yolks	2

(8 g)	Amount
Natural / soy-nut peanut butter	0.75 TBS
Almond butter	0.75 TBS
Olive/canola Oil	0.5 TBS
Peanut/almond/flaxseed Oil	0.5 TBS
Flaxseeds, whole	2.5 TBS
Olives (rinse)	7
Low-carb Protein bars	check

www.ybyl.com

SECTION 5: APPENDIX

Your Body, Your Life™

1800 Calories, Meal & Snack Plan
[30%-protein, 50%-carb, 20%-fat]

MEALS: 450 Calories / SNACKS: half these quantities

PROTEIN

(34 g)	Amount
Lean meat	6 oz
Fish	6 oz
Chicken breast	large
Lean, low-salt lunch meat	5-7 slices
Can tuna, in water (rinse)	6 oz

(34 g)	Amount
Low-fat cottage cheese	1.5 cups
Egg whites	10
Protein drinks/bars	check
Low-sodium soy burgers	check
Tofu/soy products	check

CARBOHYDRATES

(56 g)	Amount
High-fiber vegetables/salads	unlimited
Corn/peas/carrots	1.25 cups
Baked potato,	med
Bread, whole wheat	check
Bagel	1
Pasta	1.75 cups
Rice	1.25 cups
Milk, soy/skim or 1%	40 oz
Fresh-squeezed juices	20 oz
Yogurt, low-fat, plain/vanilla	20 oz

(56 g)	Amount
Yogurt, fruit flavored	10 oz
Beans/lentils/legumes	2.5 cups
Banana/apple/pear/orange	2.5
Grapefruit	2.5
Strawberries/Blueberries	2.25 cups
Grapes	70
Plums	8
Oat meal, slow-cooked	1.25 cups
High-fiber cereals	check
Protein drinks/bars	check

FAT

(10 g)	Amount
Fat from lean meat & fish	4 oz
Creamy salad dressing	1 TBS
Cheese, sliced	1 slice
Guacamole	2 TBS
Avocado	0.25
Nuts, unsalted	15-20
Egg yolks	2

(10 g)	Amount
Natural / soy-nut peanut butter	1 TBS
Almond butter	1 TBS
Olive/canola Oil	.5 TBS
Peanut/almond/flaxseed Oil	.5 TBS
Flaxseeds, whole	3 TBS
Olives (rinse)	10
Low-carb Protein bars	check

SECTION 5: APPENDIX

2100 Calories, Meal & Snack Plan
[30%-protein, 50%-carb, 20%-fat]

MEALS: 525 Calories / SNACKS: half these quantities

PROTEIN

(39 g)	Amount	(39 g)	Amount
Lean meat	5 oz	Low-fat cottage cheese	1.25 cups
Fish	5 oz	Egg whites	8.5
Chicken breast	med	Protein drinks/bars	check
Lean, low-salt lunch meat	4-6 slices	Low-sodium soy burgers	check
Can tuna, in water (rinse)	5 oz	Tofu/soy products	check

CARBOHYDRATES

(66 g)	Amount	(66 g)	Amount
High-fiber vegetables/salads	unlimited	Yogurt, fruit flavored	12 oz
Corn/peas/carrots	2 cups	Beans/lentils/legumes	3 cups
Baked potato, med	1	Banana/apple/pear/orange	3
Bread, whole wheat	check	Grapefruit	3
Bagel	1.5	Strawberries/Blueberries	3 cups
Pasta	2.5 cups	Grapes	90
Rice	1.5 cups	Plums	10
Milk, soy/skim or 1%	48 oz	Oat meal, slow-cooked	1.5 cups
Fresh-squeezed juices	24 oz	High-fiber cereals	check
Yogurt, low-fat, plain/vanilla	24 oz	Protein drinks/bars	check

FAT

(12 g)	Amount	(12 g)	Amount
Fat from lean meat & fish	5 oz	Natural / soy-nut peanut butter	1.25 TBS
Creamy salad dressing	1 TBS	Almond butter	1.25 TBS
Cheese, sliced	1 slice	Olive/canola Oil	0.5 TBS
Guacamole	2 TBS	Peanut/almond/flaxseed Oil	0.5 TBS
Avocado	0.33	Flaxseeds, whole	3 TBS
Nuts, unsalted	18-22	Olives (rinse)	12
Egg yolks	2	Low-carb Protein bars	check

www.ybyl.com

YBYL™ Sample Fitness Programs

These programs are presented in progressive order of difficulty and effectiveness and are designed to help you create your own program. If you're just beginning a fitness program, start with either Level 1 or 2 and increase your program every two to three weeks. You may substitute a physically challenging yoga class for any cardiovascular or cardio-muscular training session.

FITNESS PROGRAMS

Your Body, Your Life™

LEVEL 1:

DAY 1
- Cardiovascular training, 30 min (low intensity)
- YBYL Stretch, 10 min

DAY 2
- Cardiovascular training, 30 min (low intensity)
- YBYL Stretch, 10 min

DAY 3 • Rest and Recovery

DAY 4
- Cardiovascular training, 30 min (low intensity)
- YBYL Stretch, 10 min

DAY 5 • Rest and Recovery

DAY 6
- Cardiovascular training, 30 min (low intensity)
- YBYL Stretch, 10 min

DAY 7 • Rest and Recovery

LEVEL 2:

DAY 1
- Cardiovascular training, 30 min (low intensity)
- YBYL Stretch, 10 min

DAY 2
- Cardio-muscular Training, 30 min (low intensity)
- YBYL Stretch, 10 min

DAY 3 • Rest and Recovery

DAY 4
- Cardiovascular training, 30 min (low intensity)
- YBYL Stretch, 10 min

DAY 5 • Rest and Recovery

DAY 6
- Cardio-muscular Training, 30 min (low intensity)
- YBYL Stretch, 10 min

DAY 7 • Rest and Recovery

Your Body, Your Life™ **FITNESS PROGRAMS**

LEVEL 3:

DAY 1
- Cardiovascular training, 30 min (med intensity)
- YBYL Stretch, 10 min

DAY 2
- Cardio-muscular Training, 30 min (med intensity)
- YBYL Stretch, 10 min

DAY 3
- Rest and Recovery

DAY 4
- Cardiovascular training, 30 min (med intensity)
- YBYL Stretch, 10 min

DAY 5
- Rest and Recovery

DAY 6
- Cardio-muscular Training, 30 min (med intensity)
- YBYL Stretch, 10 min

DAY 7
- Cardiovascular training, 30 min (med intensity)
- YBYL Stretch, 10 min

LEVEL 4:

DAY 1
- Cardiovascular training, 30 min (med/high intensity)
- YBYL Stretch, 15 min

DAY 2
- Cardio-muscular Training, 30 min (med/high intensity)
- YBYL Stretch, 15 min

DAY 3
- Rest and Recovery

DAY 4
- Cardiovascular training, 30 min (med/high intensity)
- YBYL Stretch, 15 min

DAY 5
- Rest and Recovery

DAY 6
- Cardio-muscular Training, 30 min (med/high intensity)
- YBYL Stretch, 15 min

DAY 7
- Cardiovascular training, 30 min (med/high intensity)
- YBYL Stretch, 15 min

FITNESS PROGRAMS

LEVEL 5:

DAY 1
- Cardiovascular training, 30 min (med/high intensity)
- YBYL Stretch, 15 min

DAY 2
- Resistance-Training (Lower Body), 30 min (low intensity)
- YBYL Stretch, 15 min

DAY 3
- Rest and Recovery

DAY 4
- Resistance-Training (Upper body), 30 min (low intensity)
- YBYL Stretch, 15 min

DAY 5
- Rest and Recovery

DAY 6
- Cardio-muscular Training, 30 min (med/high intensity)
- YBYL Stretch, 15 min

DAY 7
- Cardiovascular training, 30 min (med/high intensity)
- YBYL Stretch, 15 min

LEVEL 6:

DAY 1
- Cardiovascular training, 30 min (med/high intensity)
- YBYL Stretch, 15 min

DAY 2
- Resistance-Training (Lower Body), 30 min (med intensity)
- YBYL Stretch, 15 min

DAY 3
- Rest and Recovery

DAY 4
- Resistance-Training (Upper body), 30 min (med intensity)
- YBYL Stretch, 15 min

DAY 5
- Rest and Recovery

DAY 6
- Cardio-muscular Training, 30 min (high intensity)
- YBYL Stretch, 15 min

DAY 7
- Cardiovascular training, 30 min (med/high intensity)
- YBYL Stretch, 15 min

Your Body, Your Life™   **FITNESS PROGRAMS**

LEVEL 7:

DAY 1
- Cardiovascular training, 30 min (med/high intensity)
- YBYL Stretch, 15 min

DAY 2
- Resistance-Training (Lower Body), 30 min (high intensity)
- YBYL Stretch, 15 min

DAY 3
- Rest and Recovery

DAY 4
- Resistance-Training (Upper Body), 30 min (high intensity)
- YBYL Stretch, 15 min

DAY 5
- Rest and Recovery

DAY 6
- Cardio-muscular Training, 30 min (high intensity)
- YBYL Stretch, 15 min

DAY 7
- Cardiovascular training, 30 min (med/high intensity)
- YBYL Stretch, 15 min

LEVEL 8:

DAY 1
- Cardiovascular training, 30 min (med/high intensity)
- YBYL Stretch, 15 min

DAY 2
- Resistance-Training (Lower Body), 45 min (high intensity)
- YBYL Stretch, 15 min

DAY 3
- Rest and Recovery

DAY 4
- Resistance-Training (Upper body), 45 min (high intensity)
- YBYL Stretch, 15 min

DAY 5
- Rest and Recovery

DAY 6
- Cardio-muscular Training, 30 min (high intensity)
- YBYL Stretch, 15 min

DAY 7
- Cardiovascular training, 30 min (med/high intensity)
- YBYL Stretch, 15 min

LEVEL 9-10: For Men, upper body emphasis

Day 1
- Resistance-Training (Upper body A), 45 min (high intensity)
- YBYL Stretch, 15 min

Day 2
- Resistance-Training (Lower Body), 45 min (high intensity)
- YBYL Stretch, 15 min

Day 3
- Rest and Recovery

Day 4
- Resistance-Training (Upper Body B), 45 min (high intensity)
- YBYL Stretch, 15 min

Day 5
- Rest and Recovery

Day 6
- Cardio-muscular Training, 30 min (high intensity)
- YBYL Stretch, 15 min

Day 7
- Cardiovascular training, 30 min (med/high intensity)
- YBYL Stretch, 15 min

LEVEL 9-10: For Women, lower body emphasis

Day 1
- Resistance-Training (Lower Body A), 45 min (high intensity)
- YBYL Stretch, 15 min

Day 2
- Resistance-Training (Upper body), 45 min (high intensity)
- YBYL Stretch, 15 min

Day 3
- Rest and Recovery

Day 4
- Resistance-Training (Lower Body B), 45 min (high intensity)
- YBYL Stretch, 15 min

Day 5
- Rest and Recovery

Day 6
- Cardio-muscular Training, 30 min (high intensity)
- YBYL Stretch, 15 min

Day 7
- Cardiovascular training, 30 min (med/high intensity)
- YBYL Stretch, 5-15 min

YBYL™ Sample Cardio-Muscular Training Workouts

CARDIO-MUSCULAR TRAINING

INCLINE TREADMILL TRAINING:
20-MINUTES + 5 MIN WARM-UP AND 5 MIN COOL-DOWN

- Warm-up for five minutes, gradually increasing the incline and speed to 3.6 mph (women) or 4.0 mph (men). Stretch lower body for five minutes.

- Maintain a 3.6 (women) or 4.0 (men) mph pace and increase incline to an angle you can maintain for 20 minutes; start with a lower incline and increase over time. Don't hold handrails.

- On the second or third workout, go for your max; record your max. As a workout, choose an incline that's 80 percent of your max. Try to exceed your max every two to three weeks.

- Cool-down for five minutes, decreasing incline to two degrees and speed to 2.5 mph; stretch for five or ten minutes.

- To add variety and interval-train, every second or third session, do a 20-minute workout with 30-second intervals of walking at a very high incline, followed by walking for 30 seconds at a very low incline.

NOTE: Record your workouts on paper.

STAIR MACHINE:
20-MINUTES + 5 MIN WARM-UP AND 5 MIN COOL-DOWN

- Warm-up on manual setting for five minutes, gradually increasing speed. Stretch lower body for five minutes.

- Choose one of the interval programs and increase speed to a level you can maintain for 20 minutes; start with a lower level and increase gradually over time; keep your heels down as you push down on the pedals and keep your back flat (shoulders up).

- On the second or third workout, go for your max; record your max. As a workout, choose a level that's 80 percent of your max. Try to exceed your max every two to three weeks.

- Cool-down for five minutes, decreasing speed to a low level; stretch for five or ten minutes.

CARDIO-MUSCULAR TRAINING

ELLIPTICAL TRAINER:
20-MINUTES + 5 MIN WARM-UP AND 5 MIN COOL-DOWN

- Warm-up on manual setting for five minutes, gradually increasing speed and resistance. Stretch lower body for five minutes.
- Choose one of the interval programs and input your body weight.
- Increase speed and resistance to a level you can maintain for 20 minutes; alter speed and resistance as you like. The goal is to burn as many calories in 20 minutes as possible; start with a lower level and increase gradually over time; keep your heels down as you push down on the pedals and keep your back flat (shoulders up)
- On the second or third workout, go for your max. As a workout, choose a level that's 80 percent of your max. Try to exceed your max every two to three weeks; record your max.
- To add variety and interval-train, every second or third session, do a 20-minute workout with 30-second high intensity intervals followed by 30-second low intensity intervals. Record your workouts on paper.
- Cool-down for five minutes, decreasing speed and resistance; stretch for five or ten minutes.

STATIONARY BIKE:
20-MINUTES + 5 MIN WARM-UP AND 5 MIN COOL-DOWN

- Warm-up on manual setting for five minutes, gradually increasing speed and resistance. Stretch lower body for five minutes.
- Using one of the interval programs, choose a resistance level you can maintain for 20 minutes. Start with a lower level and increase gradually over time.
- On the second or third workout, go for your max; record your max. As a workout, choose a level that's 80 percent of your max. Try to exceed your max every two to three weeks.
- Cool-down for five minutes on a low manual setting; stretch for five or ten minutes.

TREADMILL - 1 MILE RUN:
20-MINUTES + 5 MIN WARM-UP AND 5 MIN COOL-DOWN

- Warm-up for five minutes, gradually increasing speed; stretch lower body for five minutes.

- On a two-degree incline, increase speed to a pace you can maintain for 1 mile; you may alter speed as you like. Start with a slower speed and increase gradually over time.

- On the third or fourth workout, go for your max; record your max. As a workout, choose a pace that's 80 percent of your max. Try to exceed your max every two to three weeks.

- Walk for ten minutes at a good pace and then cool-down for five minutes, decreasing incline to two degrees and speed to 2.5 mph; stretch for five or ten minutes.

YBYL™ Super Stretches

The YBYL Super Stretch routine consists of effective, compound, multi-joint stretches and is designed to help stretch and align your entire body in a short amount of time.

YBYL - SUPER STRETCHES

YBYL STANDING PULL STRETCH:
CHEST, SHOULDERS, HAMSTRINGS, LOW-BACK, ABS

PROPER FORM:

1. Stand up straight with your feet hip-width apart. Clasp your hands together behind you so that your arms are straight and the palms of your hands face one another and rest on your tailbone. Look straight ahead and pull your hands down and away from your body. Hold for 10-30 seconds.

2. Release the stretch and relax for a few seconds. Repeat this hand position, slowly bending forward at the waist until you feel a good stretch in the shoulders, low back and hamstrings. Allow your head to drop naturally. Hold for 10-30 seconds.

3. Release the stretch and relax for a few seconds. Repeat this hand position, slowly bending backward at the waist until you feel a good stretch in the shoulders, mid back and low back. Hold for 10-30 seconds.

TIPS / CAUTIONS:

- Only stretch warm muscles at an elevated body temperature. Keep your neck neutral and relaxed.
- A slow, sustained stretch is best. Don't bob or bounce. Don't stretch to the point of pain.
- Breathe rhythmically and focus on your breathing and extending the stretch as you exhale.

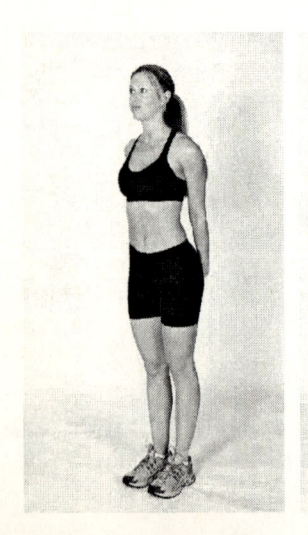

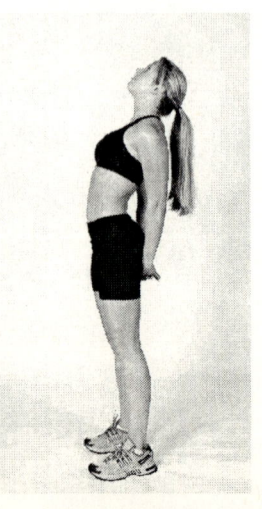

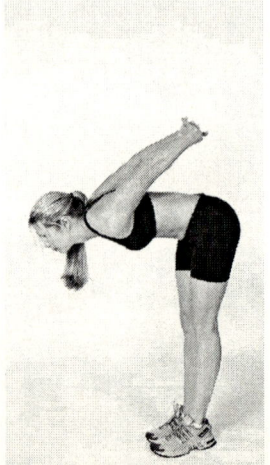

YBYL STANDING PUSH STRETCH:
BACK, SHOULDERS, HAMSTRINGS, LOW-BACK, ABS, CALVES

PROPER FORM:

1. Stand up straight with your feet hip-width apart. Clasp your hands together above your head so that your arms are straight and the palms of your hands face one another. Look straight ahead and extend your arms directly over your head as far as you comfortably can. Hold for 10-30 seconds.

2. Release the stretch and relax for a few seconds. Repeat hand position and slowly bend your upper body to the right as far as you comfortably can, while pushing your hips to the left. Keep your entire body in one plane. Hold for 10-30 seconds. Release the stretch and relax for a few seconds. Repeat stretch on other side.

3. Release the stretch and relax for a few seconds. Repeat hand position, stretching upward slowly and bending forward at the waist and stretching your hands as far forward as you comfortably can. Your legs should be straight, your hands at shoulder height and your eyes facing directly forward. Hold for 10-30 seconds.

4. Release the stretch and relax for a few seconds. Repeat this hand position, stretching upward slowly and bending forward at the waist, stretching your hands down to your feet as far as you comfortably can. Clasp your right hand under the front of you right foot and your left hand under your left foot. Bend your knees slightly if you need to and pull upward with your hands. Your chin should be slightly away from your body and your eyes should be directed between your feet. Hold for 10-30 seconds.

TIPS / CAUTIONS:

- Only stretch warm muscles at an elevated body temperature. Keep your neck neutral and relaxed.
- A slow, sustained stretch is best. Don't bob or bounce. Don't stretch to the point of pain.
- Breathe rhythmically and focus on your breathing and extending the stretch as you exhale.

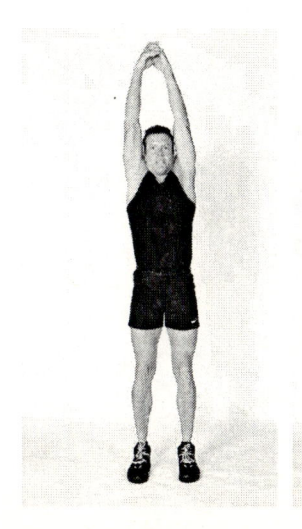

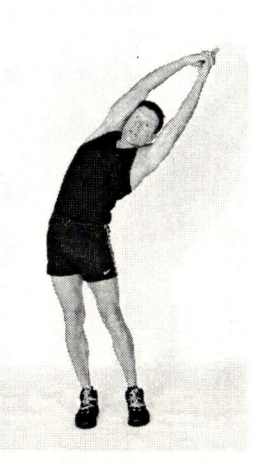

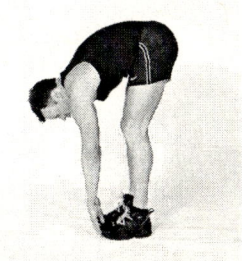

YBYL - SUPER STRETCHES

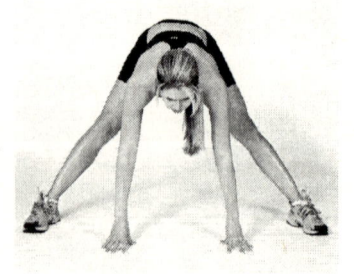

Your Body, Your Life™

YBYL SIDE LUNGE STRETCH:
GLUTEUS, HIPS, HAMSTRINGS, INNER AND OUTER THIGH, LOW-BACK, CALVES

PROPER FORM:

1. Stand up straight with your feet hip-width apart. Spread your feet outward another two feet on each side, positioning your feet at 45° angles. Keep your torso straight and look straight ahead. Slowly lunge to the right as far as you comfortably can, allowing your left leg to straighten. Place your right hand and elbow on your knee and your left hand on the floor just to the left of your right foot for stability. Keep your bodyweight on your heels and don't let your right knee extend past your foot. You may hold on to something for stability. Hold for 10-30 seconds. Release the stretch and relax for a few seconds. Repeat stretch on other side.

2. From your side lunge start position bring your feet one foot closer together on each side and rotate your feet so that they face directly forward. With straight legs or a slight bend, slowly bend forward at the waist and stretch your hands and head downward towards the floor. Hold for 10-30 seconds.

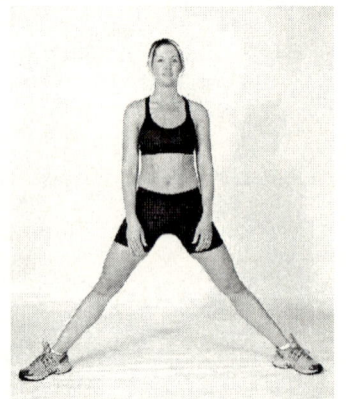

TIPS / CAUTIONS:

- Only stretch warm muscles at an elevated body temperature. Keep your neck neutral and relaxed.
- A slow, sustained stretch is best. Don't bob or bounce. Don't stretch to the point of pain.
- Breathe rhythmically and focus on your breathing and extending the stretch as you exhale.

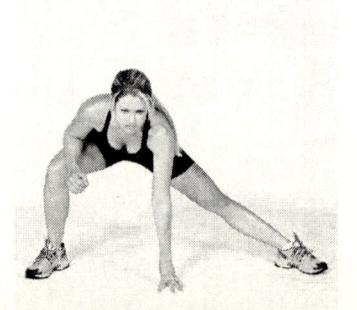

www.ybyl.com

YBYL FORWARD LUNGE STRETCH:
GLUTEUS, HIPS, HAMSTRINGS, INNER AND OUTER THIGH, LOW-BACK, CALVES

PROPER FORM:

1. Stand up straight with your feet hip-width apart. Move your right foot forward and let your left knee drop to the floor. Move your right foot forward three to four feet until it is directly over your ankle and slowly lower your left hip as far as you comfortably can. Place both hands on your right knee and keep your torso tall and straight. Hold for 10 to 30 seconds. Release the stretch and relax for a few seconds.

2. From this position, extend your right foot forward and your left knee backward as far as you comfortably can. Place your right elbow on your right leg and left hand on the floor. Allow your torso to extend forward and down towards the floor. Hold for 10 to 30 seconds.

3. Release the stretch and relax for a few seconds. Repeat the stretch on other side.

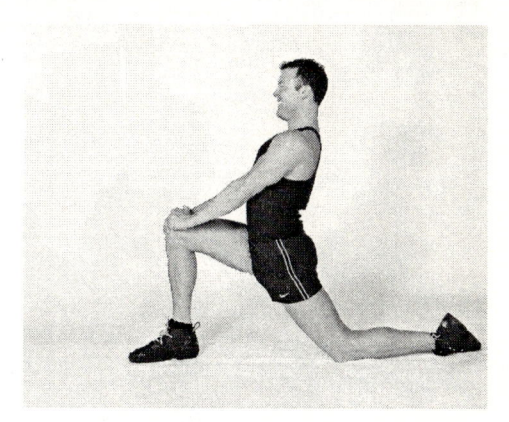

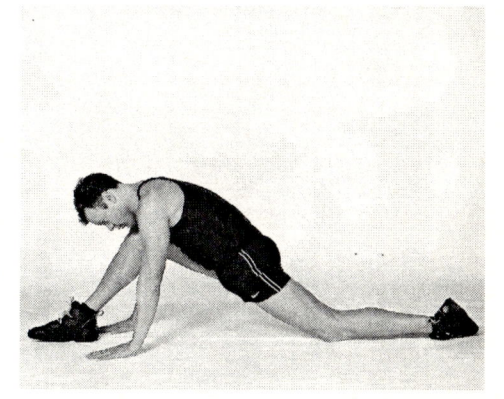

TIPS / CAUTIONS:
- Only stretch warm muscles at an elevated body temperature. Keep your neck neutral and relaxed.
- A slow, sustained stretch is best. Don't bob or bounce. Don't stretch to the point of pain.
- Breathe rhythmically and focus on your breathing and extending the stretch as you exhale.

www.ybyl.com

YBYL HAMSTRING-GLUTEUS CROSSOVER STRETCH:
GLUTEUS, HIPS, HAMSTRINGS, LOW BACK

PROPER FORM:

1. Lie on floor on your back and straighten your arms and legs. Stretch your fingers and toes in opposite directions as far as you comfortably can. Hold for 10 to 30 seconds. Release the stretch and relax for a few seconds.

2. Raise your right leg and clasp your hands over your right knee and pull your knee towards your chest as far as you comfortably can. Keep your neck and the rest of your spine flat on the floor. Hold for 10 to 30 seconds. Release the stretch and relax for a few seconds.

3. Maintain the same hand position and extend your right foot upward until your right leg is straight or slightly bent. Pull your right leg towards your head as far as you comfortably can. Hold for 10-30 seconds. Release the stretch and relax for a few seconds.

4. Place your right arm on the floor directly to your right, palm facing upward. Keep your right arm and shoulder on the floor and look to the right. Place your left hand on your right knee and slowly pull your right leg to the left directly across your body as far as you comfortably can. Hold for 10-30 seconds.

5. Release the stretch and relax for a few seconds. Repeat the stretch on other side.

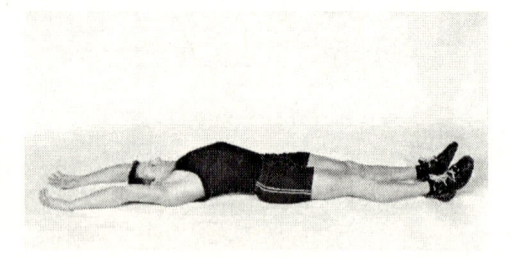

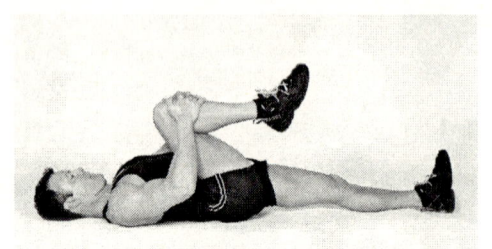

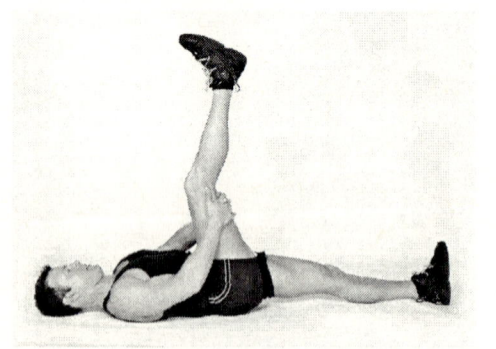

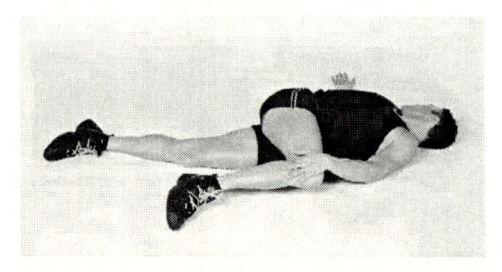

TIPS / CAUTIONS:

- Only stretch warm muscles at an elevated body temperature. Keep your neck neutral and relaxed.
- A slow, sustained stretch is best. Don't bob or bounce. Don't stretch to the point of pain.
- Breathe rhythmically and focus on your breathing and extending the stretch as you exhale.

YBYL™ Sample Resistance Training Programs

These programs are presented in progressive order of difficulty and time commitment and are provided to help you design and progress with your own program. These are only sample programs based on the YBYL resistance training exercises. If you're just beginning a resistance-training program, start with Level 1 and increase to Level 2 after four to six weeks, depending on your goals and personal preferences.

YBYL - RESISTANCE TRAINING

LEVEL 1, UPPER BODY: 30 MINUTES, 11 SETS
(WARM UP PROPERLY AND STRETCH BETWEEN SETS)

- Incline Dumbbell Press (2 sets to exhaustion, approximately 12 reps)
- Flat Bench Dumbbell Fly (2 sets to exhaustion, approximately 12 reps)
- Lat Pulldown, reverse grip (1 set to exhaustion, approximately 12 reps)
- Lat Pulldown, wide grip (1 set to exhaustion, approximately 12 reps)
- Cable Pulldown (1 set to exhaustion, approximately 12 reps)
- Upright Dumbbell Row (1 set to exhaustion, approximately 12 reps)
- Tricep Cable Pressdown (1 set to exhaustion, approximately 12 reps)
- Swiss Exercise Ball Crunch (1 set to exhaustion, approximately 30 reps)
- Romanian Deadlift (1 set to exhaustion, approximately 15 reps)

LEVEL 2, UPPER BODY: 45 MINUTES, 18 SETS
(WARM UP PROPERLY AND STRETCH BETWEEN SETS)

- Incline Dumbbell Press (3 sets to exhaustion, approximately 12 reps)
- Flat Bench Dumbbell Fly (2 sets to exhaustion, approximately 12 reps)
- Lat Pulldown, reverse grip (2 sets to exhaustion, approximately 12 reps)
- Lat Pulldown, wide grip (1 set to exhaustion, approximately 12 reps)
- Cable Pulldown (1 set to exhaustion, approximately 12 reps)
- Upright Dumbbell Row (2 sets to exhaustion, approximately 12 reps)
- Side Lateral Raise (1 set to exhaustion, approximately 12 reps)
- Tricep Cable Pressdown (1 set to exhaustion, approximately 12 reps)
- Dumbbell Bicep Curl (1 set to exhaustion, approximately 12 reps)
- Swiss Exercise Ball Crunch (2 sets to exhaustion, approximately 30 reps)
- Romanian Deadlift (2 sets to exhaustion, approximately 15 reps)

LEVEL 3, UPPER BODY OPTIONS:

If you'd like to take your upper body training program to the next level, you may consider adopting a split routine: doing all the "push" exercises on one day and doing all the "pull" exercises on another day, preferably with a 72-hour recovery period in between. If you do this, you might consider adding additional sets and exercises to each workout.

YBYL - RESISTANCE TRAINING

LEVEL 1, LOWER BODY: 30 MINUTES, 10 SETS
(WARM UP PROPERLY AND STRETCH BETWEEN SETS)

- Seated Leg Press (3 sets to exhaustion, approximately 15 reps)
- Pushback Dumbbell Lunge (1 set to exhaustion, approximately 15 reps each side)
- Side Lateral Dumbbell Lunge (1 set to exhaustion, approximately 30 reps each side)
- Hamstring Curl (2 sets to exhaustion, approximately 15 reps)
- One-Leg Standing Toe Press (1 set to exhaustion, approximately 15-20 reps each side)
- Reverse Crunch Hip Thrust (1 set to exhaustion, as many as you can)
- Back Extension (1 set to exhaustion, approximately 20 reps)

LEVEL 2, LOWER BODY: 45 MINUTES, 16 SETS
(WARM UP PROPERLY AND STRETCH BETWEEN SETS)

- Seated Leg Press (3 sets to exhaustion, approximately 15 reps)
- Dumbbell Squat (2 sets to exhaustion, approximately 15 reps)
- Pushback Dumbbell Lunge (2 sets to exhaustion, approximately 15 reps each side)
- Side Lateral Dumbbell Lunge (2 sets to exhaustion, approximately 30 reps each side)
- Hamstring Curl (2 sets to exhaustion, approximately 15 reps)
- One-Leg Standing Toe Press (1 set to exhaustion, approximately 20 reps each side)
- Reverse Crunch Hip Thrust (1 set to exhaustion, as many as you can)
- Hanging 90 Degree Leg Raise (1 set to exhaustion, approximately 30 reps)
- Back Extension (2 sets to exhaustion, approximately 15 reps)

LEVEL 3, LOWER BODY OPTIONS:

If you'd like to take your lower body training program to the next level, you may consider adopting a split routine: training lower body with certain exercises on one day and other exercises on the next day, preferably with a 72-hour recovery period in between. If you do this, you might consider adding additional sets and additional exercises to each workout. You may also add lower body cardio-muscular training to your routine, with at least a 48-hour recovery period in between.

YBYL™ Resistance Training

SWISS EXERCISE BALL CRUNCH
ABS AND OBLIQUES

This is my favorite crunch because the ball fully supports the spine and increases the range of motion. This is a great ab isolation exercise with an upper ab emphasis. However, because you must stabilize your body, it also works the serratus anterior and internal/external obliques.

PROPER FORM:

1. Sit on the ball with feet flat on floor. Lean back on the ball, making sure your low and mid back are fully supported. Bend your knees at a 90-degree angle and widen your stance for balance.
2. Gently clasp your hands behind your head, keeping your neck in line with the rest of your spine.
3. Contract your abs and lift your upper torso 3-4". Slowly lower yourself to start position. Repeat.
4. 1 rep should take about one second. When you can do 30 reps, progress to weighted dumbbell crunch. Do 1 to 3 sets.

TIPS / CAUTIONS:

- Only use your abs; keep the rest of your body relaxed and your low back against the ball at all times.
- Your hands should only be used to support your head and shouldn't assist with the crunch.
- Breathe rhythmically, inhaling on the way down and exhaling on the way up.

VARIATIONS:
Swiss Exercise Ball Crunch with a Dumbbell
Hold a dumbbell on your lap with both hands. As you walk your feet forward to push your low back against the ball, raise the dumbbell above your upper chest. Your arms should be straight, but not locked. Crunch the dumbbell up 3-4". When you can do 30 reps, increase the weight. Do 1-3 sets.

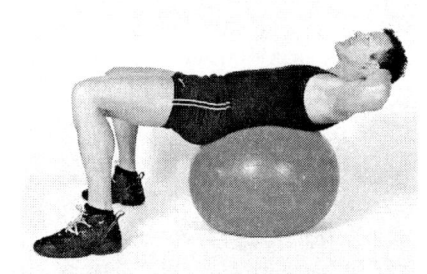

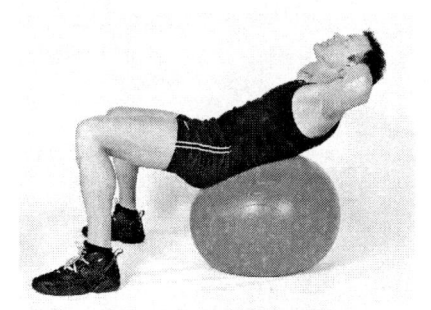

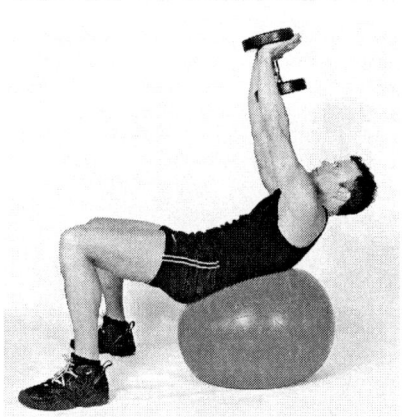

Floor Crunches
Lie on a carpeted floor or a pad. Bend your knees at a 45-degree angle and plant your feet on the floor. Gently clasp your hands behind your head, keeping your neck in line with the rest of your spine. Contract your abs and lift your upper torso 2-3" off the floor. The crunches can also be done with a dumbbell. Do 1-3 sets.

ABDOMINAL EXERCISES

HANGING 90-DEGREE LEG RAISE
ABS AND OBLIQUES

This ab crunch is essentially a reverse crunch and a great isolation exercise with a lower ab emphasis. Because your abs must stabilize your body, it also works the serratus anterior and internal/external obliques.

PROPER FORM:

1. Place your feet on the platform of a Roman Chair. Keep your back against the pad and your forearms on the pads. Hold the grips with your hands, keeping your elbows close to your sides.
2. Contract your abs and raise your knees to a 90-degree angle. This is your start position.
3. Slowly raise your knees 3-4" to your chest and slowly lower them to the 90-degree starting position. Repeat.
4. 1 rep should take 1 second. When you can do 30 reps, progress to the weighted hang raise. Do 2 to 3 sets.

TIPS / CAUTIONS:

- Only use your abs; don't swing or use momentum; keep your torso straight; don't lean forward or backward.
- Keep your legs at a 90-degree angle to isolate your lower abs and reduce hip flexion.
- Keep your low back against the pad. Breathe rhythmically, inhaling down and exhaling up.
- If you have low back issues, avoid hang raises and strengthen your abs by doing crunches on the exercise ball. Stretch your low back before doing abs.

VARIATIONS: Hanging 90-Degree Leg Raises with a Dumbbell or Weighted Ball
This exercise can also be done with a dumbbell or weighted ball between your legs or slightly bent legs to increase resistance and decrease reps. This is an advanced exercise; be careful.

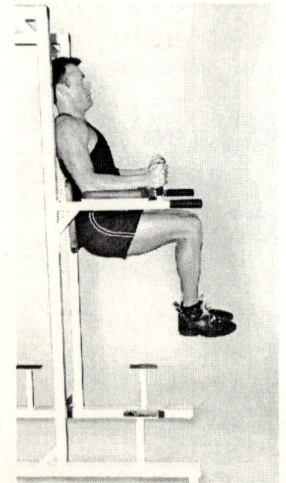

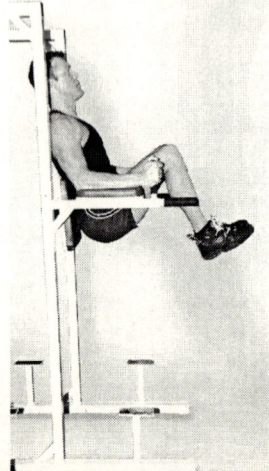

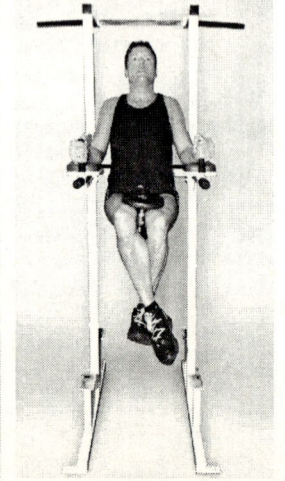

ABDOMINAL EXERCISES

REVERSE CRUNCH HIP THRUSTS
ABS AND OBLIQUES

This type of reverse crunch is a great isolation exercise with a lower ab emphasis.

PROPER FORM:

1. Lie on a carpeted floor or pad with your glutes, back, shoulders and head against the floor. Press your arms and hands (palms down) into the floor alongside your torso.

2. Slowly raise your feet 2-3" towards the ceiling, maintaining a slight bend in your knees. Your hips should rise off the mat 2-3". Your upper legs should rise up straight towards the ceiling, not angled towards your upper body. Slowly lower your legs to start position. Repeat.

3. 1 rep should take 1 second. Increase your reps until you can do two minutes without stopping. Do 1-3 sets.

TIPS / CAUTIONS:

- Focus on using only your abs; don't swing or use momentum. Put a folded towel behind your neck to support your cervical spine.

- Breathe rhythmically, inhaling on the way down and exhaling on the way up.

- If you have low back issues, avoid hip thrusts and strengthen your abs by doing crunches on the exercise ball. Stretch your low back before doing abs.

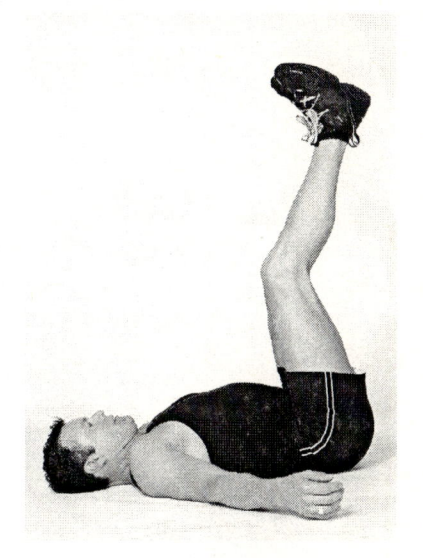

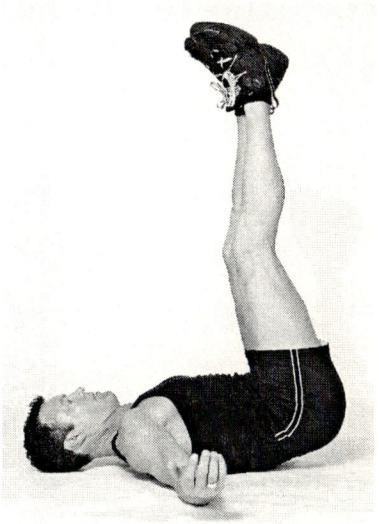

LOW BACK EXERCISES

Your Body, Your Life™

LOWER BACK EXTENSION
LOWER BACK, GLUTEUS, HAMSTRINGS, ABS

This exercise may be done on either an upper body or lower body training day.

PROPER FORM:

1. On a back extension machine, place your heels, against the metal frame of the foot platform.

2. Your quads and hips should rest against the pad so that the edge of the pad is slightly above your pelvic bone. You should be able to bend comfortably at the waist.

3. Cross your arms in front of your chest and bend forward at the waist until your torso is parallel to the ground. Keep your abs tight, upper torso up and your back slightly arched.

4. Slowly raise your head and torso until your entire spine, including your neck, is in a straight line. Slowly lower yourself to the start position. Repeat.

5. 1 rep should take 2-3 seconds. When you can do 20 reps, progress to the weighted back extension. Do 2-3 sets.

TIPS / CAUTIONS:

- Do lower back exercises at the end of a workout so that it's strong for the entire workout.
- Breathe rhythmically, inhaling on the way down and exhaling on the way up.
- Don't hyper-extend your back at the top; don't use momentum.
- If you have lower back issues or are just beginning a program, only bend halfway down. As your lower back gets stronger, progress to a full range of motion.

VARIATIONS: Lower back extensions with a barbell or dumbbell:
For advanced clients, hold a barbell or dumbbell close to your body and perform the same movement. Since the gluteus and hamstrings achieve a full contraction at the top of the movement, you may want to only bend down 4 to 5 inches to target these body parts.

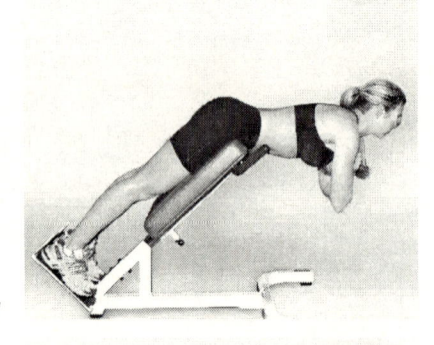

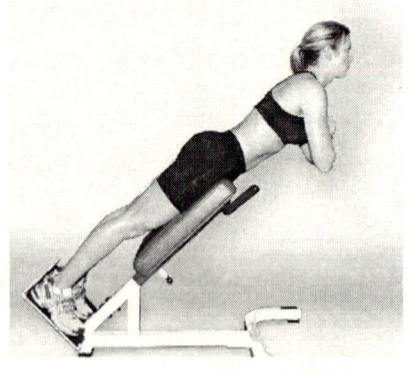

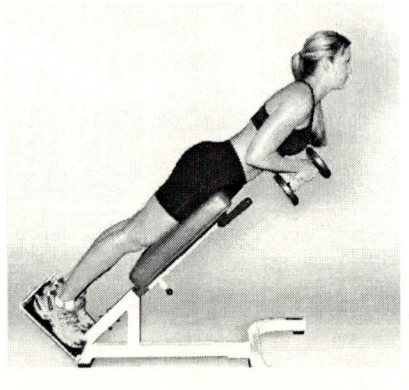

140 www.ybyl.com

LOW BACK EXERCISES

ROMANIAN BARBELL DEADLIFT
LOWER BACK, UPPER BACK, REAR SHOULDERS, HAMSTRINGS, GLUTEUS

This exercise may be done on either an upper body or lower body training day. This is one of my favorite exercises because it works so many large muscle groups. Romanian deadlifts are straight-leg deadlifts performed with slightly-bent knees that are maintained throughout the entire movement.

PROPER FORM:

1. Choose a weight that will let you maintain proper form. Position your feet hip width apart with your feet pointed straight ahead, knees slightly bent.
2. Grip the barbell with your hands slightly wider than your hips. Stand up straight with barbell against your quads; your palms should face towards your legs.
3. Bend forward at the waist until your torso is slightly above parallel to the ground. Allow your pelvis to tilt forward and stick your gluteus out and up. Keep your abs tight, shoulders up and back slightly arched. Look straight ahead. Slowly raise your body to the start position. Repeat.
4. 1 rep should take 2-3 seconds. When you can do 15 reps, increase the weight. Do 1-3 sets.

TIPS / CAUTIONS:

- Do lower back exercises at the end of a workout so that it's strong for the entire workout.
- Breathe rhythmically, inhaling on the way down and exhaling on the way up.
- Don't allow your knees to bend further than they're bent in the start position.
- Don't hyper-flex your back by allowing your head and shoulders to drop; don't use momentum.
- If you have lower back issues or are just beginning a program, only bend halfway down. As your lower back gets stronger, progress to a full range of motion.

VARIATIONS: Romanian Dumbbell Deadlifts

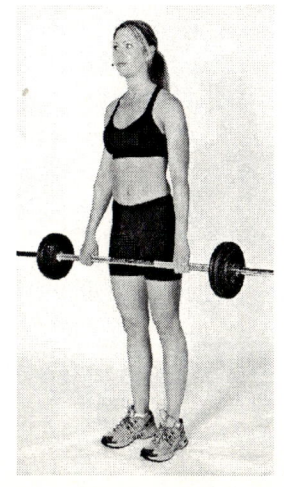

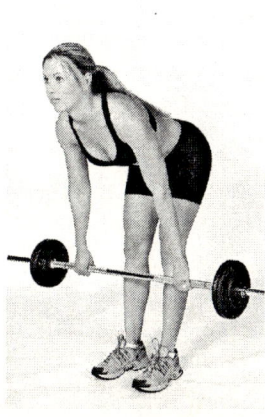

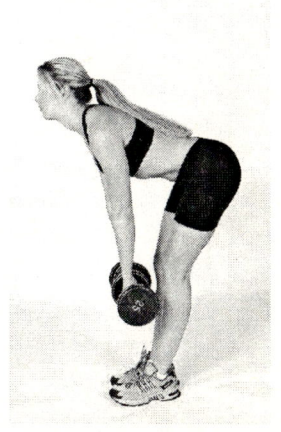

UPPER BODY "PUSH" EXERCISES

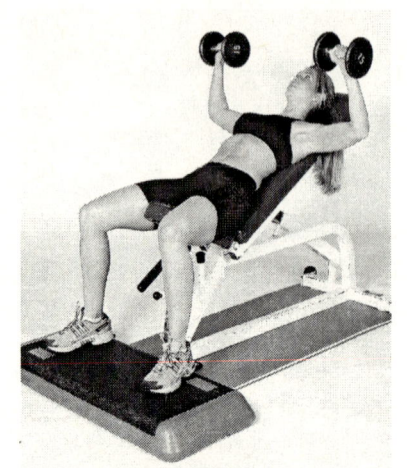

Your Body, Your Life™

INCLINE DUMBBELL PRESS
CHEST, FRONT AND MIDDLE SHOULDER, TRICEPS

This exercise targets the upper/middle chest and may be done on a flat bench. Stay within the 30-60° ranges on the bench angle. The higher the incline, the more upper chest you're working. Compared to barbell presses, these are easier to do on your own and help activate additional stabilizer muscles. Alter your arm and shoulder position to find the most comfortable lifting position. In my opinion, they're easier on the shoulder than barbell presses.

PROPER FORM:

1. Choose a weight that will let you maintain proper form. Set your adjustable incline bench to a 30- to 45-degree angle. Sitting upright on the edge of the bench, position the dumbbells on each quad just above the knee. Your feet should be wider than hip width apart and your feet should remain firmly on the ground at all times. A 90-degree angle for your knees is ideal.

2. One at a time, drive the dumbbells up with your knees so they're positioned just above and in front of your shoulders. Your palms should face forward and your elbows should point to the sides at a 90-degree angle.

3. Slowly lean back and press the dumbbells up directly over your chest, almost touching. Pause for a moment to load the muscles. Your arms should be straight, but not locked.

4. Slowly lower the weights until your elbows are just below your shoulders. Press the weights up. Repeat.

5. A complete rep should take 2-3 seconds. When you can do 12 reps, increase the weight. Do 2-3 sets.

TIPS / CAUTIONS:

- Keep your back on the bench the entire time; keep your feet on the floor. Elevate your feet slightly on a step bench if this helps your legs achieve a 90-degree angle.
- Breathe rhythmically, inhaling on the way down and exhaling on the way up.
- If you're unsure of your technique, get help from a spotter or choose a chest machine.

VARIATIONS: Flat dumbbell presses, barbell bench press, vertical chest machine, incline chest machine

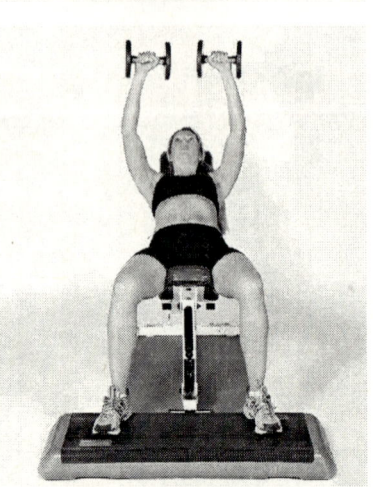

Your Body, Your Life™ **UPPER BODY "PUSH" EXERCISES**

FLAT BENCH DUMBBELL FLY
(CHEST, FRONT AND MIDDLE SHOULDER, TRICEPS, BICEPS)

This exercise targets the outer and middle chest and may also be done on an inclined bench.

PROPER FORM:

1. Choose a weight that will let you maintain proper form. Sitting upright on the edge of the bench, position the dumbbells on each quad just above the knee. Your feet should be wider than hip width apart and your feet should remain firmly on the ground at all times. A 90-degree angle for your knees is ideal.

2. Curl the dumbbells up so that they're positioned just above and in front of your shoulders. Your palms should face each other and your elbows should point to the sides at a 45-degree angle.

3. Slowly lean back and press the dumbbells up directly over your chest, almost touching. Pause to load the muscles. Your arms should be slightly bent, at about a 120-degree angle.

4. With your elbows slightly bent, slowly lower the dumbbells in an arcing motion to the side until they are parallel to the bench. Press the weights upward in an arcing motion, as if you're hugging a big tree. Repeat.

5. A complete rep should take 2-3 seconds. When you can do 12 reps, increase the weight. Do 2-3 sets.

TIPS / CAUTIONS:

- Keep your back on the bench the entire time; keep your feet on the floor. Elevate your feet slightly on a step bench if this helps your legs achieve a 90-degree angle.
- Don't let your arms go below the level of the bench and don't let your arms bend too much.
- Breathe rhythmically, inhaling on the way down and exhaling on the way up.
- If you're unsure of your technique, get help from a spotter.

VARIATIONS: Inclined dumbbell flys, pec deck machine, cable crossovers

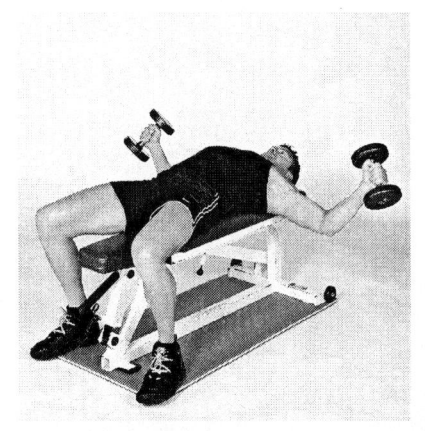

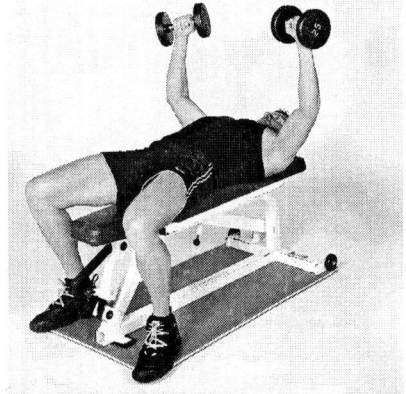

UPPER BODY "PUSH" EXERCISES

TRICEP CABLE PRESSDOWN
TRICEPS

NOTE: You're better off doing more sets of compound push movements (presses and flys) and fewer sets of isolation movements, since you're working a greater amount of muscle in the same amount of time. All chest presses performed with high intensity fatigue the triceps. I discourage one-arm isolation movements over the two-arm variety since I don't believe they are twice as effective.

PROPER FORM:

1. Choose a weight that will let you maintain proper form. Using a high-cable machine, grip a straight or slightly bent bar with a palms-down grip. Your hands should be slightly narrower than shoulder-width and your forearms should be parallel to the floor.

2. Keep your feet shoulder width apart for stability and bend your knees slightly. Keep your wrists in a locked, neutral position. Tighten your abs to stabilize your upper torso.

3. Keeping your upper arms close to your body, push the bar down toward the floor until your arms are straight, but not locked out. Let the weight slowly return to the start position. Repeat.

4. 1 rep should take 1-2 seconds. When you can do 12 reps, increase the weight. Do 1-2 sets.

TIPS / CAUTIONS:

- Do arm exercises after first completing your multi-joint, compound exercises.
- Stand tall and don't lean forward. Don't lock your knees or allow your shoulders to rise up.
- Breathe rhythmically, exhaling on the way down and inhaling on the way up.

VARIATIONS:
Dips, tricep dumbbell extensions, french presses, 2-arm tricep kickbacks.

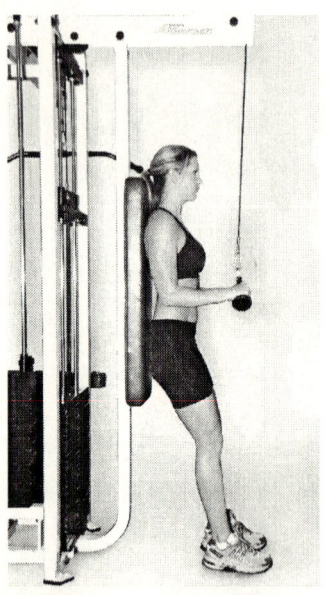

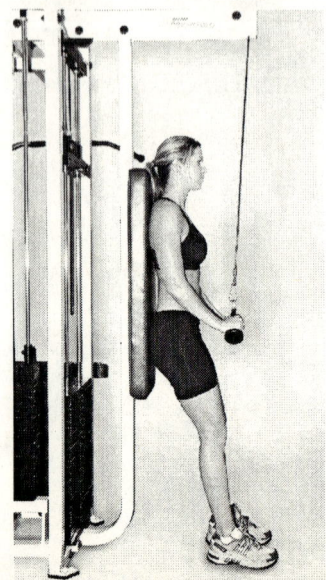

Your Body, Your Life™

UPPER BODY "PULL" EXERCISES

LAT PULLDOWN
UPPER AND MIDDLE BACK, REAR SHOULDER, BICEPS

Do these with at least two different grip positions. The reverse grip (hands face you) targets the inside of the upper/middle back, rear shoulder and biceps. The wide grip (hands face away from you) targets the outside of the upper/middle back and rear shoulders. I like the seated row a lot but it's important to use correct form so that you don't strain your lower back. I prefer lat pulls and seated rows to one-arm dumbbell rows because they work both sides of the body at the same time.

PROPER FORM FOR A REVERSE GRIP PULL-DOWN:

1. Choose a weight that will let you maintain proper form. Sitting in a lat pull machine, position your thighs firmly under the kneepads. Grasp a straight bar with a shoulder width reverse grip (hands face you).

2. Tighten your abs to stabilize your torso and arching your back slightly, pull the bar toward your upper chest until your elbows are against the sides of your torso. Let the weight slowly return to the starting position. Maintain a slight bend in the elbows in the top position. Repeat.

3. 1 rep should take 2-4 seconds. When you can do 12 reps, then increase the weight. Do 3-4 sets.

TIPS / CAUTIONS:

- Don't pull the bar behind your head on lat pulldowns; this puts too much stress on the shoulder.
- Keep your chest and chin up, but don't arch your neck too far back.
- Contract your muscles the entire time; don't use momentum.
- Breathe rhythmically, exhaling on the way down and inhaling on the way up.

PROPER FORM FOR A WIDE GRIP PULL-DOWN:

Grasp the straight bar with a hands-face-away grip 6" wider than shoulder width on each side. Follow above steps.

VARIATIONS:
Seated low row, standing bent-over barbell row, standing 2-arm dumbbell rows.

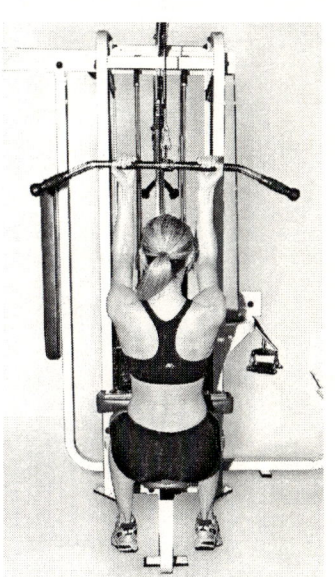

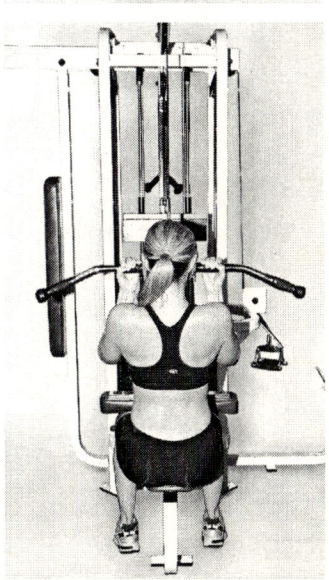

www.ybyl.com

UPPER BODY "PULL" EXERCISES

CABLE PULLDOWN
UPPER AND MIDDLE BACK, REAR SHOULDERS, ANTERIOR SERRATUS, ABS, OUTER TRICEPS

Besides targeting your upper/middle back and rear shoulders, this stabilization movement works your anterior serratus (upper ribcage muscles), outer triceps and abs. I think this is a safer exercise for most people than a dumbbell pullover.

PROPER FORM:

1. Choose a weight that will let you maintain proper form. Using a high-cable machine, grip a straight or slightly bent bar with a palms-down shoulder-width grip.

2. Keep your feet shoulder width apart for stability and bend your knees slightly. Keep your wrists in a locked, neutral position. Tighten your abs to stabilize your upper torso.

3. Keeping your upper arms close to your body, pull the bar down to your hips in an arc motion. Your arms should be straight, but not locked out. Let the weight slowly return to just above shoulder height and repeat.

4. 1 rep should take 2-4 seconds. When you can do 12 reps, increase the weight. Do 1-2 sets.

TIPS / CAUTIONS:

- Stand tall and don't hunch forward. Don't lock your knees or allow your shoulders to rise up.
- Keep a slight bend in the elbows at all times. Contract your muscles the entire time; don't use momentum.
- Breathe rhythmically, exhaling on the way down and inhaling on the way up.
- You may experiment with slight grip variations.

VARIATIONS: Dumbbell pullovers

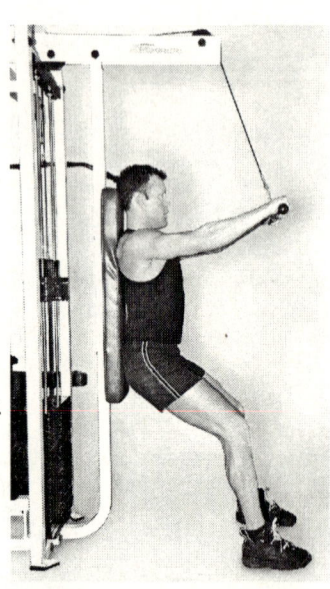

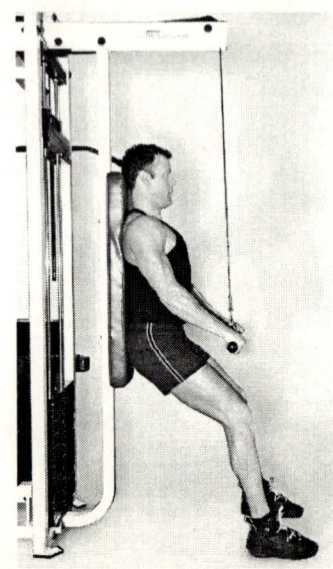

UPPER BODY "PULL" EXERCISES

UPRIGHT DUMBBELL ROW
FRONT, MIDDLE, REAR SHOULDER, TRAPEZIUS

This is my favorite shoulder exercise because, it targets the entire shoulder. It can also be done with a barbell, though I prefer dumbbells, since it allows for a greater range of shoulder motion.

PROPER FORM:

1. Choose a weight that will let you maintain proper form. Position your feet hip width apart, pointed straight ahead, knees slightly bent. Grip the dumbbells loosely with your hands, which face your body. Stand up straight with the dumbbells resting on your quads with a slight bend in the elbows.
2. Keep your abs tight and your torso up. Look straight ahead and keep your back straight.
3. Using your shoulders raise the weights up and back until they are at umbilical level and your upper arms are parallel to the ground and perpendicular to your torso. Slowly lower the weight to start position. Repeat.
4. 1 rep should take 2 seconds. When you can do 12 reps, increase the weight. Do 1-2 sets.

TIPS / CAUTIONS:

- Do shoulder exercises after first completing your multi-joint, compound exercises.
- Breathe rhythmically, inhaling on the way down and exhaling on the way up.
- Keep your back straight, head and chest up and abs tight throughout the exercise. Don't bend forward at the waist or round your shoulders.
- Keep the weights pointed down and don't raise them higher than mid-torso.
- Contract your muscles the entire time; don't use momentum.

PROPER FORM - UPRIGHT BARBELL ROW:

Grasp barbell with a hands-face-away grip slightly wider than shoulder width on each side. Follow above steps.

VARIATIONS: Upright row done with a barbell or cable machine.

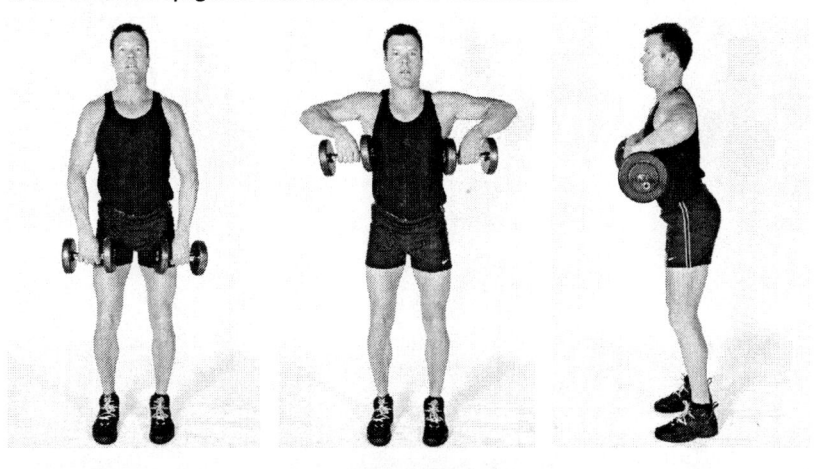

UPPER BODY "PULL" EXERCISES

LATERAL DUMBBELL RAISE
MIDDLE AND REAR SHOULDER, TRAPEZIUS

This is a good exercise to sculpt the middle and rear part of the shoulder.

PROPER FORM:

1. Choose a weight that will let you maintain proper form. Position your feet hip width apart with your feet pointed straight ahead, knees slightly bent.
2. Grip the dumbbells loosely with your hands, which are turned toward your body. Stand up straight with the dumbbells resting just outside your hips with a slight bend in the elbows.
3. Keep your abs tight and your torso up. Look straight ahead and keep your back straight. Use your shoulders to raise the weights to shoulder level. At the top position your arms and dumbbells should be parallel to the ground. Slowly lower the weight to the start position. Repeat.
4. 1 rep should take 2 seconds. When you can do 12 reps, increase the weight. Do 1-2 sets.

TIPS / CAUTIONS:

- Do shoulder exercises after first completing your multi-joint, compound exercises.
- Breathe rhythmically, inhaling on the way down and exhaling on the way up.
- Keep your back straight, head and chest up and abs tight throughout the exercise. Don't bend forward at the waist or round your shoulders.
- Keep the weights parallel to the ground and don't raise them higher than mid-torso.
- Contract your muscles the entire time; don't use your legs, raise your torso or use momentum.

VARIATIONS: Rear delt machine, front dumbbell raise

Rear dumbbell raise:
To target the rear shoulder, lean forward, arch your back and point the tip of the dumbbell slightly down at the top of the movement. These may also be done from a seated or leaning position.

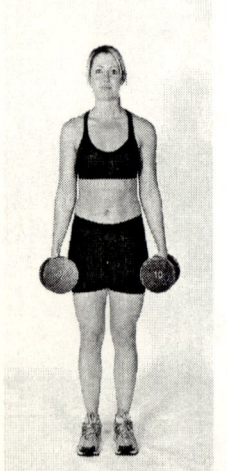

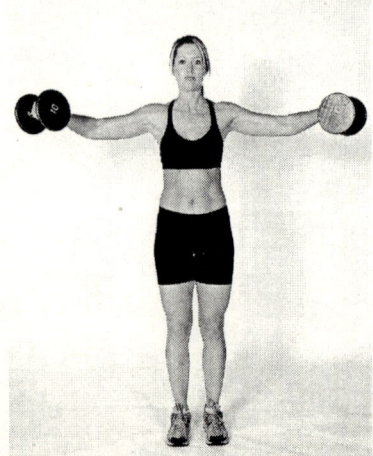

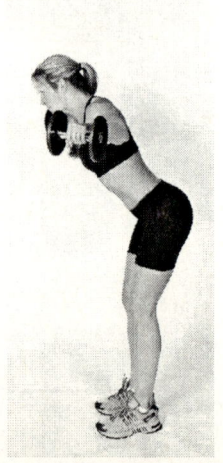

www.ybyl.com

UPPER BODY "PULL" EXERCISES

DUMBBELL BICEP CURL
BICEPS

Doing bicep curls with dumbbells helps strengthen your non-dominant arm.

PROPER FORM:

1. Choose a weight that will let you maintain proper form. Position your feet hip width apart with your feet pointed straight ahead, knees slightly bent.
2. Grip the dumbbells with your hands turned away from your body. Stand up straight with the dumbbells resting just outside your hips with a slight bend in the elbows.
3. Use your biceps to curl the weights up in an arcing motion to lower-chest level. At the top position the dumbbells should be 2-3" above your elbows and your biceps should be fully contracted, not resting.
4. Slowly lower the weight to the start position. Repeat.
5. 1 rep should take 2 seconds. When you can do 12 reps, increase the weight. Do 1-2 sets.

TIPS / CAUTIONS:
- Do arm exercises after first completing your multi-joint, compound exercises.
- Breathe rhythmically, inhaling on the way down and exhaling on the way up.
- Keep your back straight, head and chest up and abs tight throughout the exercise. Don't bend forward at the waist or round your shoulders.
- Keep your elbows at your sides the entire movement; don't allow your elbows to move.
- Don't raise the weights higher than your lower-chest.
- Contract your muscles the entire time; don't use your legs, raise your torso or use momentum.

VARIATIONS: Barbell curls, cable curls, hammer curls.

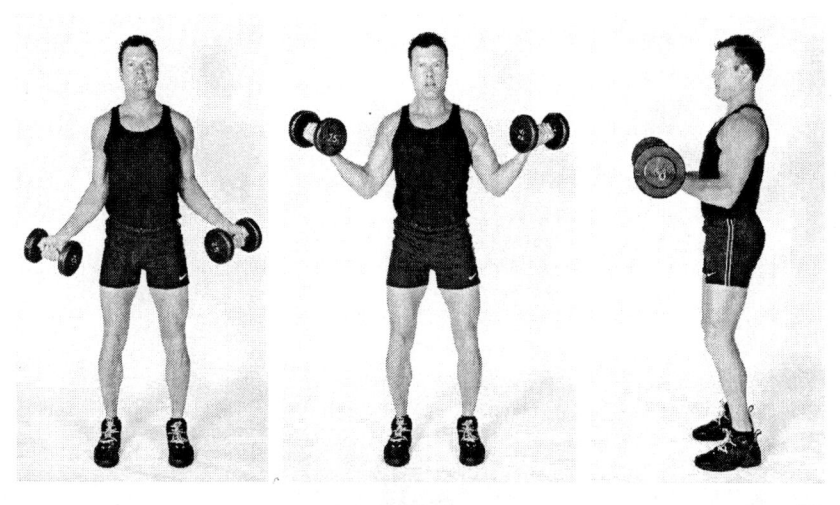

LOWER BODY EXERCISES

Your Body, Your Life™

SEATED LEG PRESS
QUADS, INNER AND OUTER THIGH, HAMSTRINGS, GLUTEUS MEDIUS, CALVES

The leg press works a lot of muscle in a very stable position. By minimizing lower back involvement, you can safely challenge yourself with more weight. After strengthening your abs and lower back, you may consider the squat. Use three different leg press foot positions. See below.

PROPER FORM (FOR THE BASIC POSITION):

1. Choose a weight that will let you maintain proper form. Warm-up with lighter weight.

2. Sit in a leg-press machine, placing your feet hip-width apart, toes pointed out slightly on the platform. Unlock the safety and release the weight. Allow your legs to bend slightly at the top position and get used to the weight. Slowly lower the weight until your legs are 90 degrees at the knee joint. Press the weight to the start position. Push from your heels, not your toes, and keep your knees slightly bent at the top. Repeat.

3. 1 rep should take 2-4 seconds. When you can do 15 reps, increase the weight. Do 3-5 sets.

TIPS / CAUTIONS:

- Keep your heels on the platform and push with your entire foot. Don't put your feet too far apart and point your toes at a sharp angle. Don't go past the 90-degree point with your legs at the bottom position. This will hyper-flex your back and may lead to injury.

- Breathe rhythmically, inhaling on the way down and exhaling on the way up.

- Keep your hips, torso and head pressed against the pad at all times. For increased back support adjust the rear pad so that it's angle is similar to the angle of the platform. Place a folded towel or pad behind your neck to support your spine. Contract your muscles the entire time; don't use momentum.

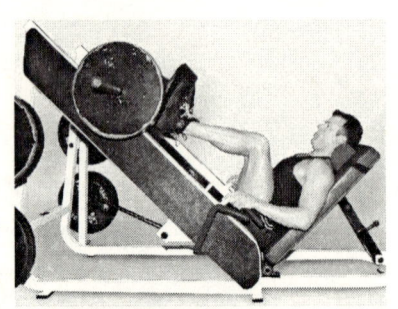

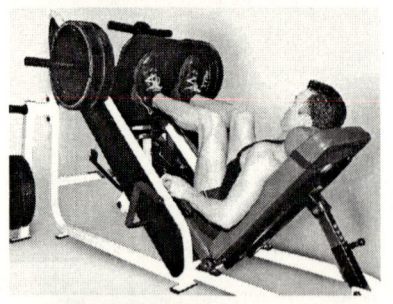

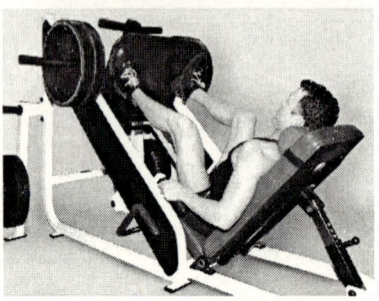

VARIATIONS: Seated Leg Press - Wide Foot Position
Place your feet 2-3" lower on the platform than in the basic position and spread them wider apart with your feet angled about 30°. This position targets the inner and outer thighs.

Seated Leg Press - High Foot Position
Place your feet 4-5" higher on the platform than in the basic power position and point them straight ahead. This position places a greater emphasis on the hamstrings.

LOWER BODY EXERCISES

DUMBBELL SQUAT

QUADS, INNER AND OUTER THIGH, HAMSTRINGS, GLUTEUS MAXIMUS AND MEDIUS, CALVES

Although the squat is a great exercise and works a lot of muscle, it is an advanced movement. Don't do these until you've spent at least six weeks strengthening your lower back.

PROPER FORM:

1. Choose a weight that will let you maintain proper form. Warm-up with lighter weight.
2. Grip two dumbbells with your hands, which are turned toward your body. Stand up straight with the dumbbells resting just outside your hips. Position your feet hip-width apart and point your toes out slightly.
3. Bend your knees and allow your pelvis to tilt forward so your gluteus is out and up - like you're sitting in a chair. Slowly lower your body until your quads are just above 90 degrees at the knee joint. As you descend, keep your abs tight, look straight ahead and keep your shoulders up and your back slightly arched. Don't let your knees extend past your toes.
4. Slowly raise your body to the start position. Push from your heels, not your toes, and keep your knees slightly bent at the top. Repeat.
5. 1 rep should take 2-4 seconds. When you can do 15 reps, increase the weight. Do 3-4 sets.

TIPS / CAUTIONS:

- Keep your heels on the ground and push with your entire foot. Don't put your feet too far apart or point your toes at a sharp angle.
- Don't lean forward too much or you'll put too much stress on your low back. Don't go past the 90-degree point with your legs at the bottom position or let your knees extend past your feet.
- Breathe rhythmically, inhaling on the way down and exhaling on the way up.
- Contract your muscles the entire time; don't use momentum.

VARIATIONS: Barbell squat.

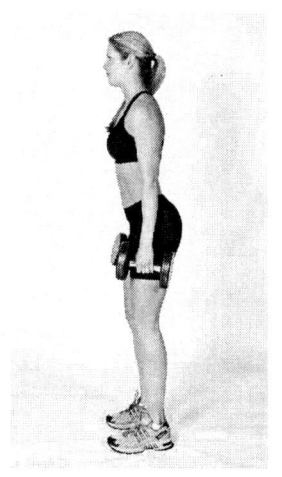

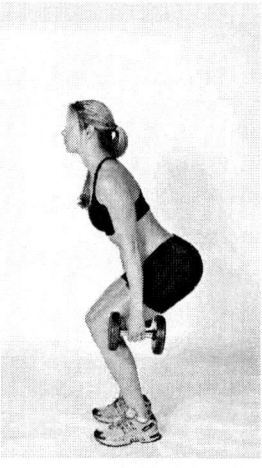

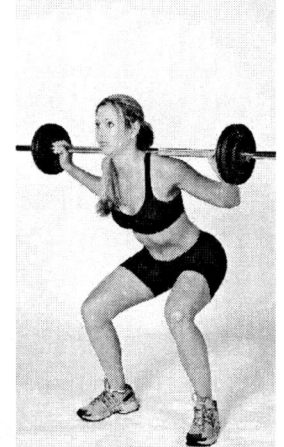

LOWER BODY EXERCISES

PUSHBACK DUMBBELL LUNGE
QUADS, HAMSTRINGS, GLUTEUS MAXIMUS AND MEDIUS, CALVES

This is my favorite leg exercise because of the muscles it targets and because it's a great functional, stabilizing movement. My clients do three types of lunges: stationary, pushback and traveling — all of which target the muscle in a slightly different way. Lunges can also be done with small, pulses at the bottom to further target the glutes while minimizing quad involvement.

PROPER FORM:

1. Choose a weight that will let you maintain proper form. Warm-up with lighter weight.
2. Grip two dumbbells with your hands, which are turned toward your body. Stand up straight with the dumbbells resting just outside your hips. Position your feet hip-width apart.
3. Step forward with your right foot. Bend at your knees and lower your hips until your left knee is a few inches off the floor and your right knee is just above 90 degrees. Push back to the start point with the right leg.
4. As you descend, keep your abs tight, look straight ahead and keep your shoulders up and your back straight. Don't let your knees extend past your ankles.
5. After you've done the planned number of reps for the right leg, rest, repeat for left leg.
6. 1 rep should take 1-2 seconds. When you can do 15 reps, increase the weight. Do 1-2 sets.

TIPS / CAUTIONS:
- Keep your heels on the ground and push with your entire foot. Don't point your toes in or out.
- Don't lean forward too much or you'll put too much stress on your low back. Don't go past the 90-degree point with your legs at the bottom position or let your knees extend past your ankles.
- Breathe rhythmically, inhaling on the way down and exhaling on the way up.
- Contract your muscles the entire time; don't use momentum.

VARIATIONS: Traveling dumbbell lunge, stationary dumbbell lunge, dumbbell step-ups

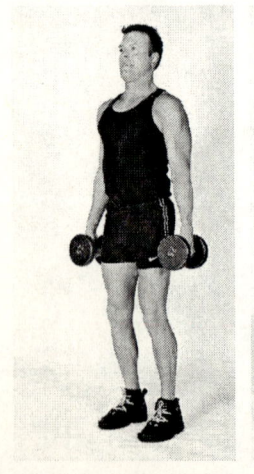

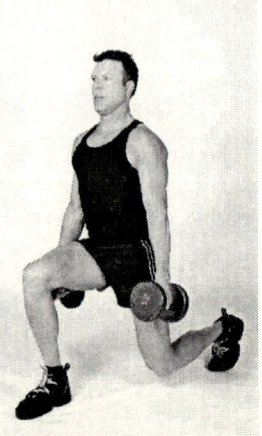

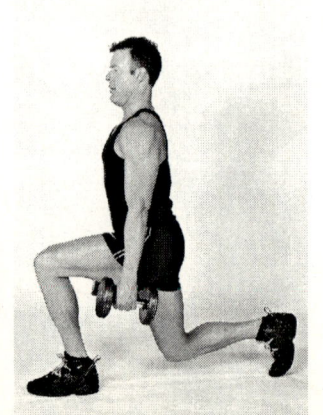

LOWER BODY EXERCISES

SIDE LATERAL DUMBBELL LUNGE
QUADS, INNER AND OUTER THIGH, GLUTEUS, LOW-BACK

This lunge, which targets a lot of muscle, can also be done with small pulses at the bottom to further target the gluteus, while minimizing quad involvement.

PROPER FORM:

1. Choose a weight that will let you maintain proper form. Warm-up with lighter weight.
2. Place a dumbbell on the floor directly below you. Spread your feet until they are about four feet apart. Open your feet so that they're at a 45-degree angle.
3. Grab the dumbbell with both hands and stand up straight. Keep your head and shoulders up and your low back slightly arched.
4. Bend your right knee and move your torso to the right until your right leg is just above 90 degrees at the knee joint. As you descend, keep your abs tight, look straight ahead and keep your shoulders up and your back slightly arched. Don't let your knee extend past your ankle. Push back to the start point with the right leg.
5. After you've done the planned number of reps for the right leg, repeat for left leg.
6. 1 rep should take 2-3 seconds. When you can do 30 reps, increase the weight. Do 1-2 sets.

TIPS / CAUTIONS:
- Keep your heels on the ground and push with your entire foot.
- Don't lean forward too much or you'll put too much stress on your low back.
- Don't go past the 90-degree point with your legs at the bottom position or let your knees extend past your ankles (try a wider foot position).
- Breathe rhythmically, inhaling on the way down and exhaling on the way up.
- Contract your muscles the entire time; don't use momentum.

VARIATIONS: Plie squats, inner and outer thigh machine, leg press or squats with wide foot position

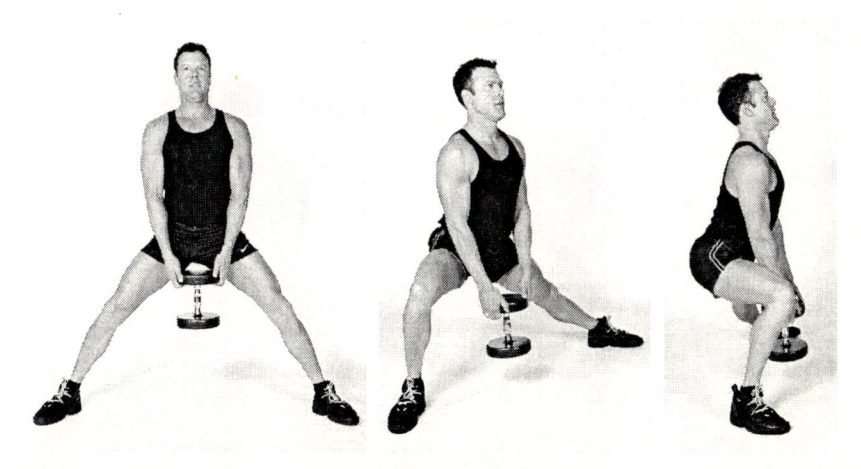

LOWER BODY EXERCISES

Your Body, Your Life™

LYING HAMSTRING CURL
HAMSTRINGS, GLUTEUS, CALVES

The hamstrings are often neglected and weak hamstrings are a major cause of knee injuries.

PROPER FORM:

1. Choose a weight that will let you maintain proper form. Warm-up with lighter weight.

2. Lie face down on a leg-curl machine and line your knee joints with the cam of the machine. Check to be sure the machine is adjusted so that the pads are resting on the back of your ankles. Press your hips down onto the pad and hold on to the handles below.

3. Slowly contract your hamstrings and raise the pad until your legs reach the 90-degree point at the knee joint. Slowly lower the weight in a controlled motion back to the starting position.

4. 1 rep should take 2-4 seconds. When you can do 15 reps, increase the weight. Do 2-3 sets.

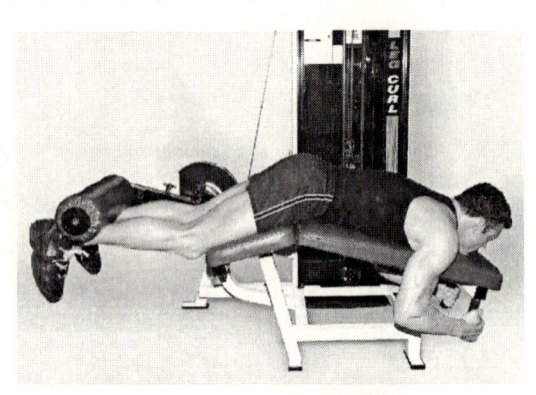

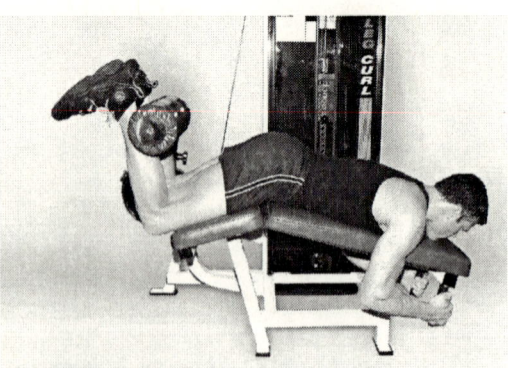

TIPS / CAUTIONS:
- Keep your hips and upper thighs on the bench the entire time. Don't let them rise up!
- Don't lock your legs out at the bottom position.
- Breathe rhythmically, inhaling on the way down and exhaling on the way up.
- Contract your muscles the entire time; don't use momentum.

VARIATIONS: Seated hamstring curl

www.ybyl.com

Your Body, Your Life™ **LOWER BODY EXERCISES**

ONE-LEG STANDING TOE PRESS
CALVES

This is easy to do anywhere and can be done with a dumbbell or with just your body weight.

PROPER FORM:

1. Stand with the ball of your right foot resting on a step or sturdy block. Hold on to something with your left hand for balance. Lift your left foot up and hook it behind your right ankle.
2. Lower your right heel as far as you can, stretching your calf at the bottom. Then press up on your toes as far as possible, contracting the calf muscle.
3. Repeat until you've done the planned number of reps for the right leg and then do the same for the left leg.
4. 1 rep should take 2-3 seconds. When you can do 20-25 reps, hold a dumbbell in your hand to increase the resistance. Do 1-2 sets.

TIPS / CAUTIONS:

- Breathe rhythmically, inhaling on the way down and exhaling on the way up.
- Contract your muscles the entire time; don't use momentum.

VARIATIONS: Seated calf machine, standing calf machine

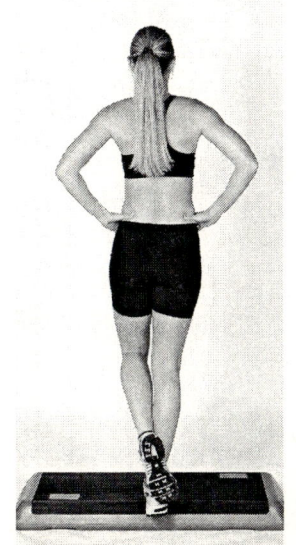

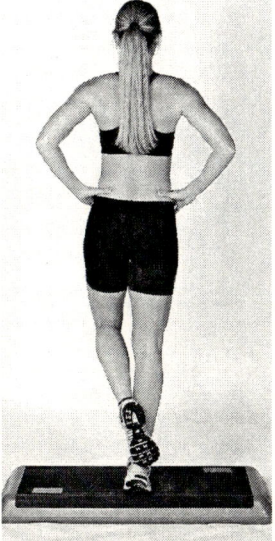

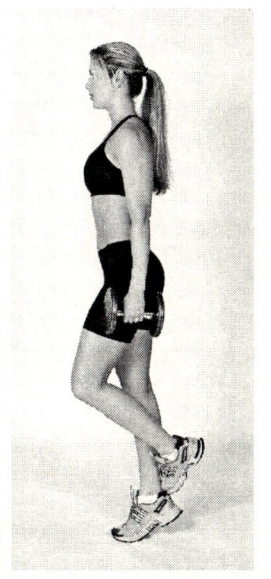

www.ybyl.com

UPPER BODY - TRAINING FORM   *Your Body. Your Life™*

YBYL - Upper Body Resistance Training Form

GOALS				DATE	
UPPER BODY EXERCISES	WT x REPS	WT x REPS	WT x REPS		WT x REPS
UPPER BODY EXERCISES	WT x REPS	WT x REPS	WT x REPS		WT x REPS
UPPER BODY EXERCISES	WT x REPS	WT x REPS	WT x REPS		WT x REPS
UPPER BODY EXERCISES	WT x REPS	WT x REPS	WT x REPS		WT x REPS
UPPER BODY EXERCISES	WT x REPS	WT x REPS	WT x REPS		WT x REPS
UPPER BODY EXERCISES	WT x REPS	WT x REPS	WT x REPS		WT x REPS
UPPER BODY EXERCISES	WT x REPS	WT x REPS	WT x REPS		WT x REPS
UPPER BODY EXERCISES	WT x REPS	WT x REPS	WT x REPS		WT x REPS
UPPER BODY EXERCISES	WT x REPS	WT x REPS	WT x REPS		WT x REPS
UPPER BODY EXERCISES	WT x REPS	WT x REPS	WT x REPS		WT x REPS
UPPER BODY EXERCISES	WT x REPS	WT x REPS	WT x REPS		WT x REPS
UPPER BODY EXERCISES	WT x REPS	WT x REPS	WT x REPS		WT x REPS
ABS					
ABS					

LOWER BODY - TRAINING FORM

YBYL - Lower Body Resistance Training Form

GOALS				DATE	
LOWER BODY EXERCISES	WT x REPS	WT x REPS	WT x REPS	WT x REPS
LOWER BODY EXERCISES	WT x REPS	WT x REPS	WT x REPS	WT x REPS
LOWER BODY EXERCISES	WT x REPS	WT x REPS	WT x REPS	WT x REPS
LOWER BODY EXERCISES	WT x REPS	WT x REPS	WT x REPS	WT x REPS
LOWER BODY EXERCISES	WT x REPS	WT x REPS	WT x REPS	WT x REPS
LOWER BODY EXERCISES	WT x REPS	WT x REPS	WT x REPS	WT x REPS
LOWER BODY EXERCISES	WT x REPS	WT x REPS	WT x REPS	WT x REPS
LOWER BODY EXERCISES	WT x REPS	WT x REPS	WT x REPS	WT x REPS
LOWER BODY EXERCISES	WT x REPS	WT x REPS	WT x REPS	WT x REPS
LOWER BODY EXERCISES	WT x REPS	WT x REPS	WT x REPS	WT x REPS
LOWER BODY EXERCISES	WT x REPS	WT x REPS	WT x REPS	WT x REPS
LOWER BODY EXERCISES	WT x REPS	WT x REPS	WT x REPS	WT x REPS
ABS					
ABS					

www.ybyl.com